Grief Before Death

A TRUE LOVE STORY

STEVIE DAHMS

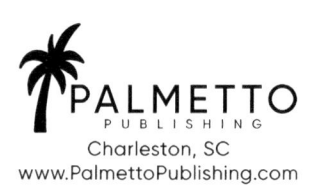

PALMETTO
PUBLISHING
Charleston, SC
www.PalmettoPublishing.com

Grief Before Death A True Love Story
Copyright © 2023 by Stevie Dahms

All rights reserved

No portion of this book may be reproduced, stored in a retrieval system, or transmitted in any form by any means—electronic, mechanical, photocopy, recording, or other—except for brief quotations in printed reviews, without prior permission of the author.

Paperback ISBN: 979-8-8229-2777-3
eBook ISBN: 979-8-8229-2778-0

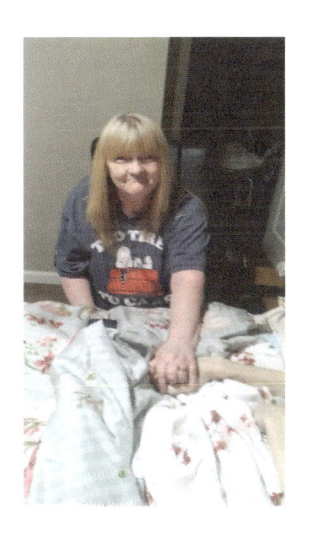

Table of Contents

Chapter 1   God Brings Them Together · 1
Chapter 2   Trials and Adventures · 8
Chapter 3   Until Death Do Us Part · 15
Chapter 4   My First Brush With Death · · · · · · · · · · · · · · · · · · 18
Chapter 5   Death And Tragedy Strikes Again · · · · · · · · · · · · 22
Chapter 6   Time For A Change · 27
Chapter 7   Warning Signs · 31
Chapter 8   Covid and Cancer · 34
Chapter 9   My Near Death Experience · · · · · · · · · · · · · · · · · · 41
Chapter 10 A Turn for the Worse · 47
Chapter 11 Dead People · 54
Chapter 12 Beginning of the End · 58
Chapter 13 Going Down the Rabbit hole · · · · · · · · · · · · · · · · 63
Chapter 14 Not Even Death Can Keep Us Apart · · · · · · · · · · 68
Epilogue · 74

Chapter 1

God Brings Them Together

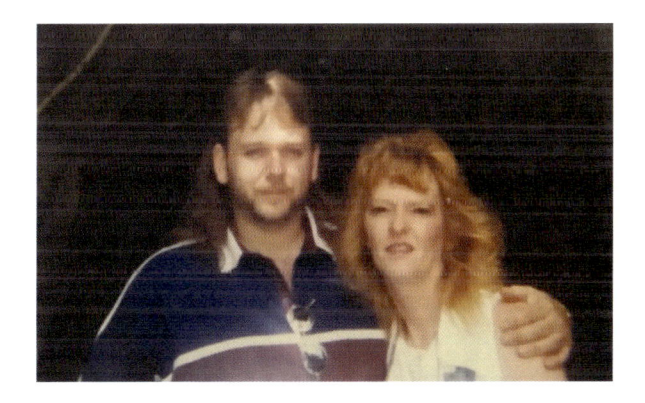

To start our story we first have to go back in time. Our story actually begins 2/27/1995 when I had a career ending injury on my job. I was an employee of the Covington IRS, and on that date the back of my chair broke causing me to land flat on my back! Out of mainly embarrassment I at first said I was OK.

The accident occurred a few minutes before lunch when I raised my hands to stretch. But by the time we got back from lunch I was beginning to feel the pain. I was able to finish the day and slowly walked home.

By the time I walked to work the next morning I was in horrible pain! My manager sent me to the nurses' station who advised me to go home and make a doctor's appointment. I was instructed to fill out an injury report and a workers compensation report. My manager asked my friend

Rochelle if she would give me a ride home. Rochelle was more than willing to take me home.

Rochelle gave me a ride to my family doctor's office, and I wasn't satisfied with his diagnosis of a strained muscle so I asked for a referral to the chiropractor. The chiropractor after the exam and x-rays said that I was done. I was beginning to fall behind on my bills and wasn't receiving anything from the IRS! Even though I lived in a section 8 apartment which paid my rent, it didn't pay my other bills! I tried hard to find employment but with chronic back injury and the ongoing workers compensation claim, nobody would give me a chance!

I was born and raised in Covington, KY and I knew that when hard times come knocking, and your back was against the wall God will step in to guide you. I also knew there was many ways to hustle a dollar, so I decided to apply at Venus, a local strip club.

It wasn't exactly my dream job I'd hoped but it would pay the bills. It would help feed my two kid's and that's what mattered the most.

The night before I was going to start my new job I prayed to God. I thanked him for blessings and asked him for understanding in my decision with the job.

I explained it wasn't what I wanted to do, and that I wasn't looking to work there for anything more than honest pay! I had already had two failed marriages and had been a single parent for a long time. I asked God to send me someone special if He saw it in my best interest.

I was nervous as I walked into the club. Since I'd been in there the day before I already knew how close to being naked you could be without going to jail. I used the name Stevie for my stage name after my favorite singer Stevie Nicks.

My friend and I liked going to the psychic fairs and having readings done. I met a lady named Debbie who told me that I was going to meet a man who was younger than I am and described him to me. She explained to me that we would become a couple and our relationship would last a long time. I could only hope she was right.

On August 10th, 1996, it would be a night I would never forget. Every dancer has to dance to 3 songs of their choice. It was almost the end of the night, and I was dancing my second song when I saw this handsome younger man standing in the archway. His hair was long and brown with eyes I could just sink into. They were so beautiful you could see them through the smoke-filled room. He was looking back just as hard.

Something about him made me feel like I knew him from somewhere, like an old friend I hadn't seen in forever. I just had to meet him before the night was over. My last song was almost over and I couldn't wait to get off the stage. 'Ohh please don't let anyone else sit with you' I thought as I was getting dressed backstage. I felt like I already knew him and I haven't even met him yet.

I'm the type of girl who believes in fate, and psychic intervention, love at first sight, and people crossing paths multiple times through many lives. I already felts that connection to this handsome stranger and I haven't even met him yet.

I came out from backstage and headed straight to him. Thankfully, he was still by himself. I casually approached him using my usual line. "Hi," I said to him, "my name is Stevie, would you like some company?" He graciously gestures for me to sit down and say, "yes, I'd love some."

The waitress is right there asking him if he'd like to buy Stevie a drink which he agrees. We started talking and I found out his name is Paul, and he lives at 12th and Scott Street. The waitress returns to see if he'd like to buy me another drink and he agrees. A dancer can only sit with a customer if he's buying drinks. He's so handsome and seems very sweet, I'm thinking to myself. He's wearing a button-down shirt with the top two buttons undone. I can see that he has lots of hair on his chest. I somehow felt so comfortable with Paul that I slid my hand inside his shirt, running my fingers through his chest hair. I was getting so aroused I wish we were anywhere else but here. I wish this night would never end. Everything felt so right sitting here with Paul.

Unfortunately, every good thing has to come to an end as we heard the waitress say, "last call." He lingered as long as he could not wanting to leave. He gave me a kiss goodbye and started for the door. I watched him leave, my heart sinking. I wondered if I would ever see him again. I sure hope so. It was damn near impossible to sleep from thinking about him and his soulful eyes.

The next few days were business as usual. I couldn't quit thinking about Paul. Just to hear his soft voice, or his beautiful eyes. It's been 3 days since I met him and he's always on my mind.

Every night I watched for him to come walking in only to be disappointed. That's the way it goes in our field of work. Here today and gone tomorrow.

But, on August 13th, while onstage I looked out into the crowd and my heart skipped a beat. Paul came walking in and he had another guy with him. I was wondering if he brought him to get his opinion of me.

I went straight to his table using my usual line. Paul immediately asked me to sit with them. Paul introduced his friend as Wes who was the boyfriend of another dancer.

They hung out for a while since Paul had to go to work in the morning. I gave him my phone number in hopes we could get better acquainted outside of the club. Before they left, Paul kissed me again. I got cold chills from my head to my feet. I already knew I wanted to keep him around for as long as possible. I felt like I've known him forever and he agrees. He was sure we'd seen each other before but none of the places we mentioned matched.

Every time the phone would ring, I'd hope it was him. I thought about Paul constantly, remembering the kiss and the feelings were electrifying. I couldn't get his eyes out of my mind.

August 17th, I was hanging around the house waiting for it to be time for work. Maybe he'll come in tonight, I thought. Instead, the phone rang, and it was Paul. He was inviting me to a birthday party Wes was having at his house for his girlfriend. I explained that I wouldn't be home until after 2:30 and he said that was fine with him. He said he would come and pick me up.

I was the first one ready to go home at closing time. I was anxious to see him outside of the club. I got home and changed into something sexy but casual. I need to put my earnings in a safe place since I was leaving. He had to bring Wes and Destiny with him because she knew where I lived. I was beyond excited when I heard her knocking on my door.

I was far behind on the partying but Paul worked on getting me caught up. I had a few beers, we smoked a couple of joints and he gave me a Xanax. I met his baby brother, Jason.

Eventually, everyone disappeared somewhere leaving us alone for the first time outside of the club. We listened to music for a while and smoked another joint. I was definitely getting a buzz now. Paul set his stereo with CDs, and he took me to his bedroom. It was the best night of my life.

Everything was perfect. I can honestly say it was the most satisfying night I had ever experienced.

We fell asleep with his arms wrapped around me. Wes woke us up to smoke an eye opener. I needed to go home because Mom would be bringing the kids home and I needed to be there to let them in. I didn't want to get out of the car, and he wasn't ready for me to either. He kissed me goodbye, and I watched him leave.

All I could do was think about him. I kept wondering why he hasn't called me yet. I'd told my friend Trina everything about him, and us. I started crying and she asked me why I was crying? I said I was afraid it was just a one-night stand. Trina replied, "If he's anything like you say it was, it wasn't." She asked me to be patient that it would work itself out.

During the course of the next week, I would get John to walk to his house with me. Paul lived on the third floor in a security building, and I wasn't able to access entry to see him. I would stand outside and throw rocks at his window in hopes he would hear it trying to get his attention. I left a couple of notes on his car telling him that I was thinking about him.

It's been almost a week since I saw him. I wasn't quite sure what to think? My Mom had just picked up the kids because they stayed with her on the weekends while I worked. Not long after they left, I heard a knock on my door, I also live in a security building, so for someone to be knocking on my door was strange. When I opened the door, to my surprise, Paul was standing there. I was so excited to see him I grabbed him and gave him a big hug and kissed him. He seemed to be enjoying that. He hung out for a while until I had to go to work, and he gave me a ride.

Today is August 23rd, 1996, and our relationship is just beginning. The night came and went, and I couldn't wait for it to be over. I just wanted to go. Right about the time I got home Paul showed up. I was so happy to see him. We went upstairs and talked for a while before I took him to my bed. After making more beautiful memories together and getting even closer to each other, we fell asleep in each other's arms.

Paul had some errands to do but asked me if I would like to go see the movie Twister with him Sunday. I've been wanting to see it, so I gladly accepted his invitation. I sat there waiting for Mom to bring the kids home because I didn't work on Sundays – that was family time. We decided to take a bus and go see it.

August 25th, 1996, I woke up in a great mood. The kids and I had a great day yesterday and Paul was coming over today. Plus, I was going to introduce him to my kids. Since I had seen Twister yesterday, he didn't think I would want to see it again, but he was wrong about that. We went out to dinner and then we went to the movie. Paul spent the night again. I was getting used to him being here with me. I just kept falling deeper in love with him.

Paul had to go to work today and the kids had school, so I had the day to myself. It gave me some time to think. Things have been slow at work, not many customers were coming in and that makes for a long night. Besides that, believe it or not, I really am an old-fashioned kind of girl. I don't think it's right to be in a relationship and out dancing almost naked in the club. I wouldn't like it!

Paul stopped by before I had to go to work and smokes a couple of joints with me before giving me a ride to work. When he dropped me off, he said he would be home the rest of the night. We kissed goodbye and went our separate ways. I went to the dressing room and started getting ready to make some money.

Everyone seemed so moody, plus it wasn't exactly hopping in there. I can only hope that will change or it's going to be a long night. But, after a few hours and only a few customers, I decided to quit. It was a hard decision, but I think it's the only one that makes sense to me. I gathered all of my belongings and walked to Paul's house. Luckily, the door was unlocked.

We had the house to ourselves and made long, passionate, love. Damn, we were so into each other, and it was electrifying when we climaxed together. He dropped me off on his way to work the next morning.

When Paul gets off work, he goes to his house and takes a shower, grabs clothes for the next day and comes to my house. He had basically been living there ever since he showed up August 23rd. It felt so right to us. It almost felt like we've walked this road before, just in a different lifetime. The connection was so strong. People could look at us and see the intensity of our love for each other. The sparks we felt when we touched was enough to burn you. But, when we made love, the pleasure and closeness was beyond measure. The love was there, and we both knew it, but it was still unspoken by either one of us.

Both of us were the oldest as far as siblings went. We both watched our parents' marriages end up in divorce. We both had failed relationships and we were afraid to admit our true feelings to each other, although we both felt the same way. I guess when the time is right, we'll admit it and take it to the next level.

Within the next week, Paul moved his stuff in. We finally admitted our love to each other. Everything seemed to be falling into place quickly, but it seemed like it took forever to get here.

On August 31st, we got our WEBN fireworks shirts, saw The Crow 2, and then went to see 38 Special play. The next day, as a family, we went to see the WEBN fireworks. It was a nice family time for us.

It was almost time for his birthday, 28 years old. We had a nice celebration and then our first sweetest day together. He was so good to me.

We were getting along great, and we had turned into a real family. I couldn't be happier. But since I live in a section 8 apartment, I wasn't supposed to have anyone else living there, so we started looking for our own place to start the rest of our journey.

Chapter 2

Trials and Adventures

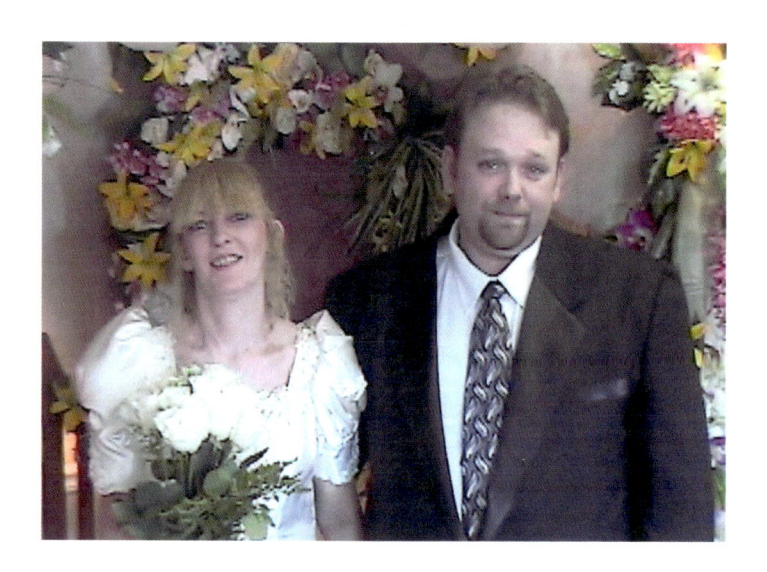

We continued to live in my apartment until November of 1997. A friend of his at his work has a two-bedroom mobile home for rent on private property so we moved to Boone County. It was small but the yard made up for it. He said I could plant some flowers since I had so much room. He said that I could get a dog too.

    I hated moving away from my mom though. She sat there and cried every day, and it broke both of our hearts. We had always lived by each other and this was the first time I had moved away from her. It would give me a chance to live closer to my dad and my sister and her family. In the long run it would turn out for the best, especially for my dad.

Paul was moving away from his Mamaw and closer to his dad as well. We both had plenty of mixed feelings about leaving them behind. We did our best to visit them as much as possible, but it still weighed heavily on our hearts and minds. We both believed in family loyalty and family comes first. We were getting used to our new place and area. Paul had grown up in that area, so he knew his way around. I on the other hand was unfamiliar to the area. Spring would be coming soon, and I was already picking out the areas for flowers and a dog.

Valentine's day was also coming up. I bought a heart shaped cake pan because I was going to surprise him with it. We *were* always big on Valentines and Sweetest days and this year would be no exception for us. We usually did flowers, cards, dinner, and gifts.

I made him the cake and decorated it. I then hid it in the oven until after dinner. When we were ready for dessert, I got the cake out of the oven and told him to come see the rest of his Valentine's day gift from me. I uncovered it and put candles on it. He walked into the kitchen, and he was so surprised when he saw it. I had written on it, and it said "Will you marry me?"

You could see the tears in his eyes as he said yes. It left us both teary eyed. We enjoyed dessert, watched TV until John went to bed. Then we celebrated the rest of Valentine's day the way we enjoyed it the best with some good sweet loving.

Paul's Mom's side of the family lives in London, KY. I met Esther in 1996, not long after we got together. Every year they had a family reunion and Paul wanted us to go with him to meet the family. We spent the night at his brother Tony's house. I met his sister Theresa who lives in Texas. We spent the weekend there and John wasn't ready to go home with us. He was having too much fun. Esther said it was OK to leave him with her so we agreed to let him stay with her.

When it came time for us to leave, I was in the kitchen with Esther and Paula, Tony's wife. She asked me how Paul and I met? I wasn't aware she already knew that and she was trying to test my honesty! I could either be honest with Esther or lie! I don't like when I'm lied to so I told her everything. She thankfully understood my position and she gave Paula a mean look. She said she was glad Paul had me and looked forward to seeing me again. Boy, was that a relief. I' m glad it was out in the open and I wouldn't have anything hanging over my head to shame me.

Wow we have a whole week to ourselves, how sweet that's going to be. I enjoyed our lovemaking much better when nobody was around who might hear us. I used to have to sleep in the same room as my parents growing up and there's things that I feel a child shouldn't see or hear. I'm glad Paul understood that. The week went by quickly and it was time for us to go to London and get John. I enjoyed Esther's company. She is a really sweet lady. We decided to play the lottery and actually won $100. Lady luck seems to be shining on us.

Today is August 14th, my 38th birthday. I'm almost 8 years older than Paul is. I already know it's going to be a good day because John goes back to school, and I have the house to myself for a while. Enjoy today because I promised Paul, I would go job hunting tomorrow.

I finally found a job August 26th at White Castle, full time, Monday through Friday and I would get home before John's school bus got there. Everything seemed to be working well for us. I wanted to save some money for Christmas and eventually our wedding.

I already had my dress. Becky, my sister, and I were at a second-hand shop and fell in love with it as soon as I seen it. Neither of us had any money though. Becky dropped me off and went to our dad s house and told him about it.

Dad called me and asked me how much it was because he wanted me to have it. It was no secret how much I wanted to be Paul's wife. Dad sent Becky to take me to the store to get the dress. I was crying I was so afraid it would be gone; my mind was full of the "what ifs"? We went straight to the wedding dresses frantically looking for it. Finally mission accomplished. I immediately put it in plastic bag and hung it up, in hopes of wearing it one day soon. August 27th, 1998 would prove to be a sad day for my family. My 2nd day on the job and I get a phone call. When I answered the phone, it was my mom, and she was crying uncontrollably. She said that my Aunt Louise, her sister had a heart attack, and they couldn't save her! I only remember sitting in the floor at work with the phone in my hand crying my eyes out. My manager asked me if I was okay and took me downstairs to the break room.

I explained to her what was going on and she said I was in no way able to drive. She was very sympathetic. Once I calmed down, she said I could go home and to keep her informed on what was going on. She said I didn't have to worry about my job. That was great news. I took the rest of the week off.

This would be the first of deaths to come to our families. Just 4 months later Aunt Louise's husband passed away. They said he grieved himself to death. Within the next year we would lose my Aunt Joan and her husband Uncle Paul, my mom's brother.

But with death comes new life. Jamie was expecting her first child. He was born August 1st, and she named him Samuel. Such an amazing day. He was so handsome.

Unfortunately, good times don't last forever. We are getting ready to go on an emotional roller coaster, and we would lose several people causing much pain and suffering.

When I met Paul, he was working for a company called Dyke building and lumber. He was a delivery driver in Ohio, Indiana, and Kentucky. Sometimes depending on his location, he wouldn't be able to receive phone calls.

It was the week of Thanksgiving 2000, and he was looking forward to having a few days off from work. I received a call from Paula, and she said that Esther had a heart attack, and she didn't make it! I couldn't believe what she was telling me, it was so sudden and unexpected.

I needed to get in touch with Paul and I wasn't looking forward to making this call. He was driving somewhere in Ohio, and I couldn't reach him. I called his boss and explained to him what was going on because they would be able to reach him to tell him to call home. Nobody wanted to tell him about his mom. Everyone knew it was going to hurt him terribly.

When he called, I was crying so he already knew something was going on. I started the conversation telling him how sorry I was and that I had bad news for him. I gave him the message Paula had told me and he just broke down crying. Needless to say, he was too upset to drive so they had to send someone to bring him back to work.

When he got home, we just held each other and cried. He needed to make a few phone calls and gather some of his clothes for the funeral. I would follow later once arrangements were made. My heart was breaking for him, and the sadness on his face hurt to see.

Esther passed away the day before Thanksgiving and nothing felt right. I made dinner for John and me, but it felt strange celebrating without him. Becky invited us to come to her house but I just needed some time to myself. Dad came and got John to go to Becky's. Dad understood that I need dome time alone. He came in and hugged me saying he was so sorry for Paul and he was crying for Paul and his pain. The look on Dad's face was the same look I would see on Paul's face. I wish I could take his pain away.

2001 is just around the corner. We hoped that the New Year would bring in a better year but no such luck. It would prove to be a rather sad time for me and my family. Tragedy would strike again, and it would put the family to their biggest challenge ever!

Dad's adventures began January 15th, 2001. I received a phone call from Dad asking me to take him to ER. He said he wasn't feeling good, and Dad isn't someone who just goes to the hospital, so I knew he was in trouble. The ER doctor said that his BP was very high and if he left, he might not make it back in time! The doctor said he would probably have a stroke. Dad reluctantly agreed to stay, and they put a call into his cardiologist. January 16th, 2001. Dad's cardiologist ordered two angiography and the results weren't in Dad s favor! They approached him about doing surgery, but Dad was still under the influence of the anesthesia.

They said all together Dad had three strokes! Dad s face was drooping, his speech was slurred, his left arm was paralyzed and also his legs. Their plan of treatment was to send him to a rehab hospital. It had just opened up.

On January 18th, 2001, Dad s cardiologist doesn't give Dad much hope. He believes Dad will continue to have strokes until he has a massive stroke which would be his cause of death. Everyone was devastated. Dad only got to be in the rehab a few days due to another stroke!

Dad would go to two other rehab facilities before being released to in home hospice April 6th 2001. Before he was released everyone had to agree on a schedule because he couldn't be left alone.

May 28th, 2001, was Memorial day. Peggy had to work so I needed to go to Dad s house. Paul and John were home waiting for me to get there. Dad didn't seem right today. The hospice nurse said it could happen at any time because Dad was tired and ready to go home.

I was tired too. I went home and made dinner and spent some time with Paul and John before falling asleep on the couch. I must've been tired because Paul said he tried multiple times to wake me up. He said we needed to go to my Dad's house and that he had passed away! What a horrible night!

But how appropriate he passed on Memorial Day. Dad was in the service but due to having drooped eyelids he wasn't allowed to serve his country. I took the rest of the summer off because I needed to get my head right. I spent summer break with John and seeing Mom as much as possible. I wanted to make sure she had her affairs in order.

With death comes new life. Isaiah Everett was born April 15th, 2002. Jamie's second son and she gave him Dad s name Everett.

Dads will says that Peggy is to be allowed to stay in his mobile home unless she decides she didn't want it, or couldn't make the payments and then I was to assume ownership. She started missing payments and with Becky's help we were able to take over the loan and pay it off.

We decided that we would be married May 24th, 2003, at justice of the peace in Covington. I wore my wedding dress, and he dressed up in his suit and tie. In attendance was his dad, Paul Sr and his wife Susan. From my side of the family was my Mom and Jamie.

After our Wedding Jamie took Mom home and she went to her house. Since we rode with his dad, we left with them. They dropped us off at our house so we could change clothes before they came back to take us to dinner.

Paul carried me over the threshold. It was a dream come true. I've been dreaming of this day for almost 7 years. Paul had always said that he would never say "I do" unless he was 100% positive it was going to last. I'm glad I get to be Mrs. Dahms for the rest of my life. Let the honeymoon begin.

We had several drinks, smoked a few joints and slow danced for a while. We eventually found our way to the bedroom and enjoyed each other thoroughly. Like fine wine it just gets better with age.

The next day Paul, John and I went to London because he wanted to introduce me as his wife to the rest of his family. It meant a lot to him to know that I was accepted into the family. We both took a week off for our honeymoon just the two of us because we took John to Mom's house. Boy ohh boy, did that week go quickly. Back to reality. Time slipped on into the future and on December, 14th, 2003, Jamie gave birth to Olivia.

Jamie had a difficult pregnancy. The doctor kept saying there was complications and wanted to abord the pregnancy all together. Jamie wasn't about to let that happen and fought as hard as she could to make sure Olivia had a chance at life.

Chapter 3

Until Death Do Us Part

Every marriage has its problems and ours was no exception to the rule. I was a sexual abuse survivor. I had trust issues, and I was very jealous. I had been betrayed by so many people who claimed that they loved me and would never hurt me. What a joke that was.

Paul liked watching pornography which only fueled my jealousy and insecurities. Like most couples we had money issues. I never won my workers compensation claim and was currently working, through temporary services. Add all that together and it was a whole lot of trouble just waiting to happen and it did!

We got a loan to pay off my student loan and a few other bills. The remainder of the money I put in the bank for emergencies. I wanted it left in the bank but he didn't see it that way! The fights became more intense, and he left me January 2005! He got his own place and told me that he loves me, but he's not in love with me anymore! Totally took me to my knees! My entire world was in shreds.

I just wanted die! I couldn't stand being away from him. All I could do was cry. I would drive by his apartment in the hopes of seeing him. I never did. I got a job through the temporary service because I had plenty of bills to pay and I was on my own now, alone, and scared.

In April 2005, Paul called me saying he wanted to come home. I was really excited to hear that but so much time has passed, and a lot of hateful things have been said to each. Could we survive it? It's definitely going to take a lot of work and patience for things to be the same again, if ever. It wouldn't take us long to get back because tragedy struck like a thief in the night!

Paul's Aunt Brenda had open heart surgery for a leaking aortic valve. She choose the pig valve but unfortunately her body rejected it. She passed away May 26th, 2005. We gathered ourselves together reeling from the news and went to London for her service. Nobody had known we had been separated and we wanted to keep it that way.

Time moves on and so did we. Every day was just another day for us. The year is now 2007.

I noticed with each passing day that I was more and more rundown. I just couldn't get enough sleep for some reason. I was working at Rally's, and it was only part time. It's not like was hard work. So, what is wrong with me? I was afraid to ask.

Paul and I seemed to have the worst luck of anyone we knew. If something was going to go wrong, it would happen to us. I had an upcoming appointment with my cardiologist and Paul thought it would be a good idea if I mentioned it to him. I hesitantly agreed.

At my appointment with Dr. Dias, I explained to him what was going on with me, and staying so tired all the time. He suggested we get some testing done and an echo done on my heart. None of which turned out good news for us. The cardiologist office called me remind me of my upcoming appointment I was instructed to bring Paul with me. That didn't sound very good to either one of. The next few days was pure hell for us. All the 'what if's' we were asking ourselves.

We were sitting in Dr. Dias office anxiously waiting for him to come in. When he came in the room, he had a serious look on his face. He explained that the echo discovered my aortic value was leaking, and I needed to have it replaced ASAP. He compared it to filling up a water balloon too full and it busting!

We never saw that one coming! He explained that I can't have any kind of infection anywhere in my body in order for it to accept the valve. I would have to get all of my teeth removed! There was too much infection in my mouth.

By this time, I'm crying my eyes out. Is this for *real*? It seemed like nightmare. This was the same surgery his Aunt Brenda had done for the same reason! I'm only 37-years-old and I'm in no hurry to die!

I was scheduled for total extraction of my teeth at UC hospital in Ohio. It seemed like it was over pretty quickly, but Paul said it took over an hour to get it over with. I was released with antibiotics and pain medication. My entire mouth hurt so bad, especially the right side.

Something didn't feel right. It felt extra swollen and thick. Even today, as I'm writing this! I never got an explanation of why.

Chapter 4

My First Brush With Death

I was referred to Dr. Gibson to discuss the aortic value replacement surgery. We saw him sometime in January 2008. He was very pleasant and brutally honest about the procedure, side effects from the valve, and what if my body rejected it. He said that we had two options as far as the valve went. There was a mechanical valve, it was called St. Jude, and the other was a pig valve. After what had happened to Brenda, we already knew it wasn't going to be that one.

They scheduled my surgery for February 27th, 2008. Just a few weeks away! I felt like I was in shock. Somebody please wake me up from this nightmare. The time went by quickly. With all the testing and paperwork, I had to do before the surgery I might as well been living at the hospital.

The night before the surgery, we brought my mom to the house. She would be going to the hospital with us. We had to be at the hospital by 5am, and the surgery was scheduled to begin at 6 am. I'm not sure if I got much sleep and I know Paul didn't. We were exhausted by the time we got there. I had my stuff packed for a few days now, just do a double check just in case I forgot something. They said I would be inpatient for a few days.

We were all so nervous when we got to the hospital. Before anything was done, I had to take a antibacterial shower for 10 minutes. I had to be thoroughly sterilized to make sure no germs could get in me, or the valve! I've had my share of surgeries in my lifetime, but this is about as serious as it can get. I'm terrified beyond belief!

Finally, they get me totally prepared for the surgery and they are going to let them come back to see me before the surgery. I have Paul, Mom, and John with me. Mom was crying uncontrollably. You could see the fear, and concern on all their faces. I was so scared, and I was crying too. The 'what ifs' really had my BP sky-high. Saying goodbye to each other was horrible. None of us knew how things were going to go in there. We were told how high risk it was and what he was going to do to me. They came in and said it was time to go to the operating room. The room was freezing cold! It felt like I was in the morgue! Dr. Gibson walks in, and he's asking me if I'm OK, assuring me I had nothing to worry about. He explained to me again exactly what he was doing to me and asked me if I understood. I nodded yes but I really didn't want to.

In order to get to my heart, he was going to have to break my sternum and for the rest of my life it would be wired shut. He would then have to take my heart out of my body. He would have to be able to keep it beating while he puts the valve in and hopefully my body doesn't reject it. *So many things could go wrong* I was thinking. It would take several hours to complete the surgery and get me to ICU.

During the surgery I had a stroke, and nobody caught it in time. Paul told me later that Dr. Gibson at one point during the surgery he had to go out and talk to him. It happened when he had my heart out and was putting the valve in! I don't remember much about my hospital stay, they kept me pretty drugged. The pillow would become my best friend. I was given a pillow to help with the pain especially when I coughed. I remember them trying to get me up to sit in the chair. I spent an extra 5 days in ICU because of the stroke.

I was released March 4th, 2008. I was so glad but also afraid to go home. I was so excited, but I was scared to leave the hospital. The what ifs was playing havoc on my mind. I would have several new medications I would have to start taking. The most important ones would be the blood thinners and the water pills. As if the valve isn't scary enough, the blood thinners could make me have another stroke! I could also bleed to death depending on my INR levels I would have to go to the anticoagulant clinic every day for a while upon release. I would have to continue with the testing for the rest of my life!

I was able to get Mom to spend another week with me. She was spoiling me, and I really enjoyed her company. We had a lot of snow since I've come home. Paul had to take Mom to her house because she was out of her medications, and we were getting a good snowstorm. I was going to have to be by myself until they get back and Paul called saying that the highway was at a standstill because of the weather. I sure hated it when she went home. I would have to try to do everything for myself and be alone while Paul was at work.

I had been sleeping in my recliner since I came home from the hospital. It was the only place I felt comfortable at because I was in a lot of pain. Since Mom went home, I had to be more mobile, and I was rebuilding my strength. I was missing sleeping next to Paul. I had tried a few times to sleep in our bed, but I wasn't ready yet. I was finally able to get comfortable enough and it felt so nice lying next to him. Another step forward.

I wasn't feeling well in April 2008. I had to make an emergency appointment with my heart surgeon's associate. I was informed that I had fluid in my lungs and on my heart! They needed me to go straight to the hospital and they would let them know I was being re-admitted. It took them several days before they could get it under control.

I was still recovering from surgery when we received news that Paul's Granny Pearl had passed away. She was Paul's granny from London. She was the most beautiful-spirited woman I had ever met. She always had good home-cooked food when we would go visit her. She passed away June 3rd, 2008. I wasn't able to travel yet so I stayed home.

I had filed for Social Security disability before the surgery just in case anything happened. Of course, it was denied but my attorney was taken care of everything for me.

John, in the meantime was expecting his first child with Catie. They were separated before Jackson was born on July 11th, 2008. We didn't get to spend much time with him. He had a head full of red hair just like my dad's. John got to see him for a few hours at Christmas time. He's such a happy baby and you can definitely tell he's Johns son because he looks just like him except for hair.

I'm grateful for how 2008 played out. So many things happened during this year. My heart surgery, Paul's granny passing away, Jackson being born and so many blessings bestowed upon us. I can only hope that next year will be better for us.

Chapter 5

Death And Tragedy Strikes Again

I don't think many people would be prepared for the hell 2009 would bring! The stock market was crashing, companies *were* closing their doors, and unemployment was at an all-time high.

Unfortunately, Paul's company would be one of those companies to fold, leaving us with very limited resources to survive.

We decided to ask Tony to move in with us to help us with bills so we wouldn't lose our home. John wasn't staying there much these days so that helped a little bit. It would be beneficial for all of us in the long run. We just didn't know what the future had in store for us.

I got sick near the end of April and my family doctor put me on antibiotics. Neither of us realized that they interfere with blood thinners! On May 2nd, 2009, I woke up with the worst headache ever! I assumed it was because of the sinus infection until I started puking up blood and couldn't stop.

Paul and Tony were building the shed so we could watch the Kentucky Derby. I asked John to take me to the ER. The MRI showed I had another stroke! The entire back of my head was filled with blood! It hurt just to open my eyes or attempt to move. I spent a week in ICU barely able to lift my head. The sound of a phone sounded like a bomb going off. We *were* definitely relieved that it wasn't worse.

In the meantime, Paul Sr. was having issues with his mitral valve leaking! He needed surgery to repair it but the closest hospital able to perform the surgery was in Minnesota! That would be a long ride for him especially after the surgery. It definitely didn't help him any! Despite all the instructions he was given he attempted to do things he shouldn't have been doing which resulted in him passing away June 23rd, 2009. It was just two days after his birthday. Needless to say, we were completely devastated.

Mamaw Ruth was suffering from dementia, loss of smell and previously had a stroke. She decided to move to a new senior facility closer to us. Paul had recently started a new job and was working second shift, so he wasn't there when she called for help. She had fallen on the kitchen floor she said when I answered the phone. I told her I was on my way, and I would call Paul to let him know what happened. Since it was assisted living facility someone was there to let me in her apartment, and she was laying on the floor. She was in a lot of pain. We called the ambulance to take her to ER in Florence. The x-rays showed her hip is broken! She would have to get surgery and do rehab therapy for a while. There's no way she can live alone now.

Surgery was a success but a couple of days later while doing therapy she fell and broke it again!! The dementia along with the sundowner syndrome they were taking over. It was horrifying to see. We had no idea how bad it was! How long has this been going on? We had no idea how much worse it was going to be either!

One night the nurses called me and asked me if I could come to the hospital because they couldn't get her to calm down. I agreed and was on my way there. It was really bad. She kept wanting to go home, trying to get out of the bed, and yelling for her mom. It took some time to get her calmed down and lots of effort. I even got in the bed with her until she fell asleep. But no sooner than I got her to sleep, Paul came in and woke her up. I was furious and left!

We brought her to live with us. It wasn't easy because of the sundowners and dementia. She tried multiple times to leave, even climbing out the front window of the trailer, with a broken hip! She didn't sleep well and would lay in bed screaming for her mom and wanting to go home. We were so exhausted, and we didn't hear her leaving one morning. The neighbors behind us found her standing in the street and called the police. We were searching everywhere for her and scared for her. The neighbors seen us looking for her and said she was in their house. Thank God. We took her home and put deadbolt locks on the door.

My heart broke for her. I loved her so much and at times we were thicker than thieves. She even liked Lil Wayne lol. I listened to rap music at that time of my life, and she liked the song 'How to Love' by him. We listened to a lot of gospel songs to and love to sing with each other. But tragedy would strike again leaving me in a deep depression I didn't think I'd ever get over.

My mom, Sarah, was the best friend any daughter could ask for. We always helped each other and the love she gave me was unmeasurable. After Dad passed away, I made sure she had life insurance, a living will and her will drawn up. Since I'm the oldest it was my responsibility to make sure that she was taken care of. She's always had her share of health issues. I'm not sure which one was the worst. She had multiple issues with her heart, (diabetes issues with her pancreas pancreatic cancers runs in the family), and circulatory issues with her legs.

The doctor unfortunately found more blockages in her legs requiring surgery. The doctor explained that if it didn't work this time the next option would be amputation. She said she would rather be dead than not be able to walk.

She would be admitted to St. Elizabeth October 19th, 2012 for stomach issues, kidney infection, and dehydration. I called her October 21st, 2012 but for some reason she could barely talk. Why? Her nurse got on the phone and said Mom had been going downhill for a little while. They were transferring her to ICU!

She suggested I call the rest of the family. I couldn't believe I was hearing this. Was she trying to tell me that my mom is dying? I think I'm in shock!

I made the necessary phone calls to the family and headed to pick John up and then to the hospital. Most of the family was already there. Before long, the doctor came out and he didn't give us much hope. He suggested that we let her go. He agreed to let Becky and myself go back to see her.

She was crying, begging me to take the tubes out because they hurt. She told us she loved us and those were the last words she ever spoke.

I was the executor of her will and living will, so I could let her go! But I didn't! The doctor gave us a small ray of hope and I prayed for a miracle. I called Paul and Brother Ellis, the pastor of the church.

Mom didn't want to be on life support, but I couldn't let her go without a chance, could I? But it was God's will for her to go home and she took a turn for the worst. I agreed to take her off life support and she passed away October 22, 2012. My life would never be the same without her. I never felt so helpless in my standing at the head of the hospital bed watching her take her last breath.

The guilt consumed me. I felt like I just killed my mom. Dear God forgive me! The feeling of guilt I'd carry was almost unbearable. I thought about suicide often but never attempted it. It would take many years and many tears to realize I had no reason to feel guilty. I let her breathe again but in heaven. I pray that I'm worthy enough to join her and all my loved ones when God says so, Jamie and Howard were working a lot so I started watching my grandkids. We were all hurting from losing Mom. I'd like to think it helped all of us.

Nothing stays the same though. My heart was about to be shattered again and I never saw it coming.

Jamie and Howard were being shuffled through temporary services sometimes because they didn't have work. They decided to move to Texas in hopes of Howard working with his dad. Jamie told me about their decision to move away and she was crying. I'm glad I was sitting down.

It felt like Mom was dying all over again, the pain was the same feeling. My beautiful Princess was moving to the other side of the world it felt like and taking my meaning to life with her. I felt so alone and heartbroken. But like everything else Paul would pull me through it. I'm so lucky to have him in my life.

Mamaw was so helpful. She showed me lots of love and understanding even as her own mental and physical health was declining. She was plagued by UTI infections, and she would literally just go out on you. After numerous visits to the ER, it was recommended that she be admitted to hospice! I went to visit as much as possible but I wasn't strong enough to stay after what I had been through with Mom. Paul never left her side except to step outside her room and smoke a cigarette. She passed away December 5, 2014. She was 94 years old. We were both grieving the loss of our loved ones, which only brought us closer than we'd ever been. We were alone a lot more than usual since John moved out and Tony worked a lot of double night shifts. It felt so great to lay in his arms, being kissed so passionately, the familiar cold chills when he would touch my body. He made me feel things I d never felt with anyone else. We weren't just having sex; we were truly making love. The kind of love you hear about, see in a good movie, or dreamed about. I feel so blessed, not just for making love to my husband, but for the real love we shared between us.

Chapter 6
Time For A Change

Another year begins and it's my birthday. I'm turning 55. The year is 2015. I'm not feeling well so Paul is making me a birthday cake. He decorates it with cream cheese icing and crumbles up cookies and puts on top of it. Not a whole lot happened in 2015 so we're going to jump into 2016. It starts out with a family emergency.

Jamie's dad Gary cut his leg pretty good. He never told anyone about it and tried to doctor it himself. Fortunately, some members of Jehovah witness stopped by his house and were able to get him medical treatment. He was taken to St. Elizabeth hospital and admitted to ICU. The wound was badly infected and was septic. The condition of his release was someone would have to live with him and take care of him. Paul wasn't working at the time so Jamie asked him if he would be interested in taking care of him.

Paul agreed and stayed with Gary for several months and he saved his life a couple of times. Gary was so grateful for everything Paul had done for him and they set his house to be transferred to him in his will and in a land contract. Gary was filing for bankruptcy and Paul loved the house and location.

February of 2016 I was admitted to the hospital to have my gallbladder removed. It was supposed to be a simple procedure but not for me. After the surgery I stopped breathing twice and they had to issue Code Blue. Absolutely scared Paul when they told him about what was happening to me.

Valentine's day of 2016 was the first time we weren't together! I was still in the hospital with a snowstorm coming! I could see the expressway from my hospital room window and traffic as a disaster! My nurse was sweet, and she came to my room and stayed with me as much as possible.

Gary was admitted back in the hospital June of 2016. The doctors weren't giving him much time to live. It was decided that he would move to Texas and live with Jamie and her family.

Paul had recently submitted his application for employment in the mobile home park we lived in, and they hired him. It couldn't have happened at a better time especially with his first house payment due. He already had tomato plants growing there and I had watermelon plants ready to be planted.

Jamie and her family came to town to help Gary get everything together for his move to Texas. It was so nice having her back home even if it was temporary. I tried to spend as much time with her as possible, I wasn't looking forward to when she would be going back to Texas.

Paul and I slowly started getting our stuff packed up and moved into the house. It was really nice to just be with each other alone. We have been together for 20 years now and this is the first time it was just the two of us. Our love got more and more intense each time we made love. I felt so comfortable, I didn't have to worry about being quiet anymore.

Our closest neighbor was up the hill, or over the other hill. Never in my life was I able to enjoy screaming with pleasure multiple times. And so many different places to enjoy each other in ultimate ecstasy. We knew each other so well we could have conversations without barely speaking a word. We were always in each other's heads even if we weren't around each other. Not many people get to be so lucky. I think it's a "Once in a lifetime" thing. We were definitely blessed to have each other.

I had multiple watermelons growing. One of my personal sized one was just beautiful inside. Perfect red color with a white sugary glaze to it, and the best watermelon I'd ever eaten. One of my watermelons weighed 27.6 pounds and I fed 5 families with it.

But summer ended and our first winter and holidays were upon us. The snow was so beautiful and heavy. He had the day off work, so we decided to play a game. We called it "snow day".

We pretended we were at my house and my parents were at work. We made love multiple times, each time more exciting and intense than the time before, I still smile just thinking about it. I'm so much in love with Paul. Thankfully he's just that much in love with me. Thank you, God, for bringing us together.

The kitchen was so small that cooking Thanksgiving dinner was a real treat. It was so worth it though when it was done. Paul always enjoyed decorating for Christmas and he was even more excited this year. There was so much more to decorate and he really went out of his way to make sure it looked nice. It wasn't long after Christmas I got a phone call from Paul telling me he's bringing chickens home! We had been talking about it, but we weren't set up yet for them yet. It was definitely an adventure because we had a dog, plus a pack of coyotes in the area. The next morning, after doing a head count, only 1 was missing. We spent the day fixing up a pen for the chickens. Since he worked a lot, it became another one of my responsibilities. It wasn't so bad until winter came, then it wasn't exactly easy to do.

Christmas day came and went, and it was New Year's Eve. We celebrated and brought in 2017.

Time moved on and soon it was the month of May. Time to get out our seeds for our gardens and get our flowers planted. It takes a lot of time and work to get it all done but the rewards were always well worth it.

We had planted onions, tomatoes, several different types of pepper, and green beans. During the day time it was my responsibility to tend to the gardens, but once he got home, and unless he had a bad day, we took care of them together. It was nice providing our own food and being able to share with family.

But my biggest surprise would come July 17th when I was feeding the chickens and saw our first egg. I almost didn't see it, but when I did, I took a picture and sent it to him. He called, immediately excited as well. The chicken started making more eggs than we needed so I started selling them to the people running the corner store at the top of the hill. They loved fresh brown eggs and were grateful to get them. It was pretty cool the way life was going for us. We felt so blessed.

Chapter 7

Warning Signs

But nothing good lasts forever, as we all know. Just when you get a few steps ahead, you get knocked back twice as far!

The year is now 2018. Gary's health was declining.

He was in and out of the hospital several times. Jamie was going to have to get surgery on her foot because of the torn ligaments. She was exhausted trying to take care of her family, the house, cooking, and working from home. Jamie's foot was terribly swollen from not being able to rest it like she should.

Meanwhile, Gary was released to "in home hospice". He sadly passed away December 24th, 2018. I heard the phone ringing and ran downstairs to answer it. It was between 1-1:30 am, Jamie was crying and telling me that he had went home to Heaven.

The rest of 2018 was depressing, and I was glad it was over! I can only pray that 2019 will be more productive and pleasurable.

But 2019 would prove to be a strange year of unexplained events. Little did we know that they were the "Warning Signs" of things to come.

For some reason, Paul started hearing a woman's voice out of nowhere while he was sleeping. He swore it was me yelling for him and he could still hear it after it woke him up. She was yelling his name and nothing else. He would start yelling for me and asking me what I wanted. I didn't have a clue what he was talking about!

I started noticing a change in his appetite and how quickly he became tired. Sometimes he was going be to bed at 8-8:30! Just out of the blue he would get up and say he was too tired and go to bed! Even if Tony was there and they were playing PlayStation! This isn't natural for him to do.

Paul wasn't the only one hearing voices. Just out of the blue I was hearing a man's voice saying my name. Of course, I would assume he was yelling for me, and I would go upstairs to see what he needed. He would still be sleeping when I went to ask him if he yelled for me! The voice I heard reminded me a lot of my dad's voice. Then the dreams started, strange dreams that I found to be alarming! In my dreams we were sleeping, and I would roll over to hug him, but he had passed away. I would freak out, crying, screaming, and yelling. I would then call Tony and tell him that Paul had passed away in his sleep! Tony would be on his way to the house, but before he got there, I died too! Then, I would wake up. I was so scared because the dream seemed so real that I would rub his body until he spoke. What a relief it was to hear his voice.

Paul always drank a lot of water and Mountain Dew. I would notice in the middle of the night upon going to the bathroom that his urine had a foul odor to it. He never complained like he had any kind of infection going on, so I let it drop. But the more time went by, the stronger it became. It had gotten to the point that I actually puked a few times from the odor of it. The house used a water pump that would run if you didn't jiggle the handle just right.

One day, we were casually having a conversation about things in general, and the conversation turned to his health. We started discussing how his appetite had changed, how fatigued he was, the smell of his urine and how dark it was becoming. He informed me that he had trouble being able to urinate recently. Out of nowhere he states that he was pretty sure he had cancer! I couldn't believe he was saying that about himself. It was rather alarming to think about!

It was almost time for his 6-month health checkup. I told him to make sure to let Christina know what was going on and see what she could do to help him. He chose not to mention it because he was worried, he would have to take a drug test and we smoked marijuana.

As we approached the end of 2019, nothing or nobody could prepare us for what 2020 was going to bring!

Chapter 8

Covid and Cancer

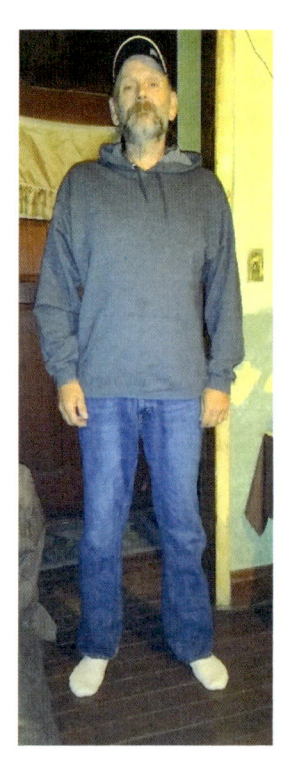

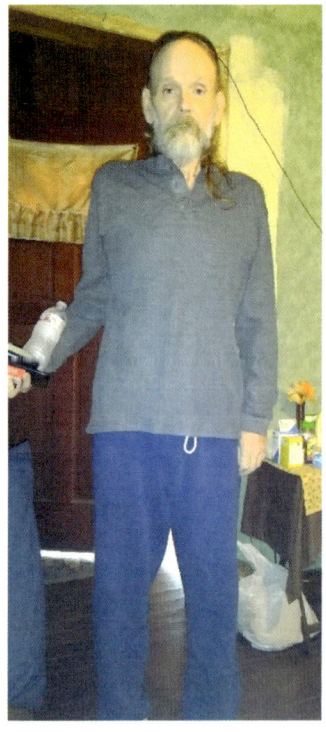

2020 came in like a lion and never let go of its grip!

It was so cold and snowy. It's getting harder for Paul to chop the wood and get it into the house for the burn barrel. Good thing I got up early and could get it going again. So far, he hasn't had many snow days yet, but on the days he did, we definitely made more memories. We both had been sick recently, and we both were diagnosed with a sinus infection. The antibiotics seemed to help us, but it took longer to get better.

Then, in March of 2020, President Trump announced that a virus had been reported in China! Many people were sick and dying! It was a fast-spreading virus called Covid 19! On March 11th, it was declared a Pandemic. The world was placed on lockdown! Since it is an airborne virus, everyone has to wear a mask! Our world as we had known it is gone forever! I admit it was beyond depressing! I would listen to the news updates, and the daily afternoon updates from our Governor Beshear and just sit and cry.

Paul could see how badly it was affecting my mental health. I decided to make him a Dallas Cowboys blanket to keep my mind occupied. It was going to be a wedding anniversary gift, but I couldn't wait until then. He absolutely loved it and was truly surprised when he saw it. It wasn't easy keeping it hidden from him and the only time I could work on it was when he was at work.

He was sick longer than I was, and our family doctor gave him a referral to see a lung doctor. The lung said that he has lung disease and the beginning of emphysema. He wasn't like this before he got sick. Did he have Covid instead of a sinus infection?

With my health the way it was, Paul didn't want me going out to the stores or anything. He would call every day before coming home from work to see if we needed anything. May 12th, Paul was getting out of his truck and coughed at the same time. He said that the pain was so intense, he was sure he had broken his rib! I don't think I've ever seen him in so much pain! We contacted our doctor, and she ordered a chest x-ray.

May 13th, 2020, our entire world came crashing down on us! He had his chest x-ray done that morning and Christina called him a few hours later. She explained to him that there were no broken bones, but there were some pulmonary nodules! She was crying and explained to him it meant he had cancer! She said she was going to send him for a CT scan, and it would be able to tell her more. She ordered it STAT! It was scheduled for May 15th. Christina called rather quickly with worse news! The CT scan showed too many pulmonary nodules to count! They needed to do another CT scan which was already scheduled for that afternoon! The news was that he would have to go see an oncologist ASAP! All we could do was cry in total shock!

Since we were still in the Pandemic, no visitors were permitted in the doctor's office or the hospital! He was starting the beginning of his biggest fight ever completely alone as far as medical treatment goes. I felt horrible for him. As much as he went through with me and my health, and I couldn't be there for him. The first time he gets sick, it's a matter of life and death and I can't be by his side every step of the way!

Paul started seeing oncology in the end of May 2020. Since I couldn't go in with him, he would set his phone on speaker so I could at least listen to what was being said while I sat in the car waiting for him. Dr. Sapp explained to him that he was being diagnosed with Stage 4 metastatic RCC, clear cell carcinoma. There is no cure! The first step of treatment was to make a doctor's appointment with the urologist to have surgery to remove his right kidney and gallbladder ASAP.

I took a picture of Paul on May 20th, 2020. He had already lost a lot of weight. On May 20th, a full bone scan was done. Our 17-year wedding anniversary was coming up and since everything was shut down due to Covid, we would be celebrating at home. It was May 24th. We shut out the whole world! We turned off our phones and tried to enjoy the day as best as possible. Before he got up, I blew up 18 balloons. I hung the extra one in the living room and I told him it was for next year, crying the entire time. I was trying to give us both hope for our future. I fixed a nice dinner, but he didn't have much of an appetite, understandably. God bless his heart and soul.

Everyone in the family was concerned for Paul, for both of us. A lot of them were concerned as to what I would do when he passed away. I had always told everyone that I couldn't imagine 1 minute without him. If he died, I wanted to die, too! He was worried about me as well and made me promise that I wouldn't do anything to hurt myself when it happened! Jamie would call me every day making sure I was OK, trying to keep me focused on living, especially after the dream I had been having! Becky talked to me multiple times, crying with me, and asking if there was anything we needed. We definitely needed a new mattress, especially with how fast he was losing weight. Rochelle and I would talk on messenger multiple times a day, plus all our phone calls to each other. Theresa was always talking to us through text and the phone. Tony was by our side basically daily. To be honest, I don't know what we would have done without him. I started calling us The Three Amigos. It definitely described us. Becky, in the meantime, had told Jamie, Mandie, and Leah that she was raising money to help us out with a new mattress. She placed the order and Jamie was asked to let us know when it was going to be delivered so we would be home to accept it. We just cried, especially Paul. He was deeply touched by the gesture of love they showed us. It was delivered June 9th, 2020.

Between Paul's upcoming surgeries, radiation, testing, and the narcotics he was prescribed, he had to resign from his job. Kevin, the owner of the company, wouldn't accept it and instead laid him off. At least that way he could get unemployment! Because of the pandemic and Kentucky unemployment computers being so old they shut down; Paul wouldn't see any of it for over a year!

When Paul went to his first appointment with the urologist, it was terribly hot outside, so he parked under a big shade tree so I wouldn't get hot. Like any other doctor appointment, he had his phone on so I could listen in. When he explained to Dr. Dusing what I was doing, Dr. Dusing instructed me to come to his office! He didn't follow that rule and he agreed that I needed to know what he was planning on doing. He would be removing Pauls' right kidney, and the surgery was schedule for June 19th, 2020. A different doctor would be removing his gallbladder, and a robot would be used to help with the procedure.

Tony spent the night the night before, and we took Paul to the hospital. It was horrifying watching him go in by himself. He's such a good man who doesn't deserve any of this! We sat there and watched him until we couldn't see him anymore before we drove away. We were tired when we got back to the house, but our anxiety was more dominant. We were definitely worrying about Paul. The doctor said he would call after the surgery was done. We finally heard from the doctor, and everything went according to plan. Paul was in recovery. He explained that the gallbladder was badly diseased and that it had turned porcelain! The hospital was only allowing 1 visitor at a time, but I couldn't see him until tomorrow. That sounded like an eternity to us.

He was able to call once he got to his room. It was nice to hear his voice. He was in a lot of pain. They were only giving him Tylenol for his pain. He gave me a list of things he wanted me to bring him. He said that the catheter was really bothering him. Once we hung up, I immediately called the nurse's station. I explained to them his medical condition, and I gave them a complete list of his medications, which included morphine and oxycodone! There was no reason for him to be in pain! I instructed them to give him his medications or I would call every one of his doctors! He called me back saying that the nurse just came in and him his pain medication. They apologized because they were unaware that he had pain medicine for his cancer. I just acted surprised and was definitely relieved. Now he doesn't have to hurt anymore!

He was released June 23rd. Since it was raining, I asked Tony to pick him up. That way, I wouldn't have to fight with the driveway. I started a GoFundMe account since he still hasn't heard anything from unemployment. Our only income was my Social Security check for $649! We can't live on that!

June 24th, we got the biopsy report stating that it was clear cell carcinoma! On June 25th, he would be starting a series of radiation treatments. Dr. Sapp started him on Keytruda and Cabozantinib. The Cabozantinib he was prescribed to take 1 a day for 21 days and then skip a week. Then he would be done with them. If only things went the way they were supposed to, right? By the time Paul finished radiation therapy, he had lost even more weight! He was more fatigued, but he was still trying to do things that he used to be able to do. It was heartbreaking to see, but I couldn't take his pride and dignity away from him. Paul would do 6 weeks of radiation before his surgery and another 6 weeks after the surgery. He started taking the Cabozantinib and 1 chemo treatment July 13th. On July 21st, his port was placed in his chest to make it more convenient for all the testing and treatments he would be receiving.

But, August 11th, he couldn't get enough to drink, pounding bottles of water and immediately puking. He kept getting weaker and he was trembling. I went against his wishes and called Dr. Sapp. I was instructed to take him to the ER, but he refused to go. I begged and pleaded with him to go with the same results. I called Tony and explained to him what was happening. He came to the house and by the time he got there, Paul was a mess! He wanted to walk outside to sit and clear his head. He almost passed out at the table! We got up to go inside and he was so wobbly Tony had to help him inside. He was trying to convince us he was OK, but when we got inside, he almost passed out again! Tony basically had to dress him so that we could take him to the hospital. Especially since Dr. Sapp had her office call since he hadn't been to the hospital yet! They had called the hospital to let them know that he was coming in to be checked out.

Tony had to go with us because Paul was still puking and couldn't walk! They took him back immediately. He had a garbage bag full of green vomit!

Thankfully, he had a port in because they ordered multiple vials of blood be drawn! The nurse noticed a "fruity odor", finger nail polish remover smell on his breath! She said it was DKA! His labs confirmed what she said was accurate. His blood sugar was 1057! I learned that smell and it was a good thing because it happened multiple times! It destroyed his pancreas and now he has stage 1 and 2 diabetes. His potassium level was sky-high. He could've died! Paul was admitted into the ICU where he would stay for the next 6 days!

My birthday was August 14th and I spent most of the day in the hospital with him. The catheter was really bothering him, and he was upset because he didn't get to do anything for my birthday. I assured him that was the least of my worries. I cried all the way home. It was the first time in 24 years that I would spend my birthday alone.

Jamie called me and talked to me for a while. She sent me some money for my birthday, and I went and got myself some dinner. I don't know what I would do without her.

The doctors concluded that the Cabozantinib was what caused everything to happen to Paul and he was told to stop taking it.

Our 24-year anniversary as a couple was August 23rd, 2020. It has always seemed like we've known each other much longer, especially with everything we've been through. We locked out the whole world again and spent a peaceful day with just the two of us.

We were looking forward to the next day because John was coming to visit us. It's been a long time since we last saw him. He was going to go to Texas to live with Jamie for a while. It was hard on John to see Paul like that.

On August 20th, Tony and I had to take Paul back to the hospital. His BP was very low, and he was puking again, and very pale He was in shock! He was admitted back to ICU and released 2 days later.

But what was coming next for us would take everyone by surprise! It would leave me fighting for my own life and him scared to death that I was going to die before him! He always said if anything ever happened to me that he would crash the truck off of a cliff!

Chapter 9

My Near Death Experience

One of my favorite things to do is to listen to music. We were always introducing each other to music we hope the other one would like. He played a song for me called "Until Then" by Zulle Erna. We just sat and cried.

I was sitting outside one morning, smoking a joint, trying to be quiet and talking to Theresa on the phone. Out of the corner of my eye I saw a glimpse of something bright. I turned to look at it full force and to my surprise it was what I can only describe as an Angel! I gasped and Theresa asked me if I was okay. I started telling her about it.

She (he, because Angel's are male from what I was taught) was beyond anything I had ever seen in my life! Her hair was long and blonde, the dress she was wearing was not from our world! It was long and seemed to float in the breeze.

Such a bright light surrounded her

I started crying, thinking she was there for him. I don't think Theresa knew what to think about what I was telling her. Then, just as fast as she appeared, she was gone even faster.

I told Paul and Tony about it. Paul had a strange look on his face, and he asked me if I told her that he wasn't ready yet. I told him I didn't have time to say anything to her because she disappeared. We would find out soon enough who she was there for.

August 30th, I just wasn't feeling well. My right leg was really bothering me, and I was beginning to run a fever. I basically slept the entire day.

You know I'm sick when I don't even want to smoke a joint. I even slept downstairs because it hurt me to try and walk upstairs.

I felt horrible the next day and I sent a message to Christina via MyChart. I explained to her what was going on and how my mom had all those blockages in her legs. She advised me to go to the ER to make sure I was OK. It wasn't what I wanted to hear. I was scared, not just for myself, but for Paul. What if I had to stay? Who would be there for him?

When we got there, I was feeling horrific. When they found out that Paul had cancer, he was made to go to the car and wait there for his safety. Things were spiraling out of control! Suddenly, my fever shot up to 105.6! I needed to pee, but I wasn't allowed to walk to the bathroom, so they had to bring a portable potty in for me to use. I was texting Paul, Jamie, and Theresa keeping them informed on everything. When I was done urinating, there was a drop of blood, and my leg was really red and burning. I started feeling like I was going to puke but spit up blood instead! The nurse went to find the doctor.

Nobody knew what to think when I was texting them about the blood and I sent them pictures as well. I was texting Paul when suddenly I couldn't breathe! I started banging the tissue box on the bedside table, and I think I said I couldn't breathe to the nurse, and I don't remember anything after that!

Yesterday was September 1st when I went to the ER. Today is September 2nd and I was up in the ICU! My entire right leg was bandaged from my toes to my thigh. I couldn't talk.

The nurse explained that I had a tube in my throat, and I couldn't talk yet. I had no idea what had happened to me or where I was except, I was in the hospital! I kept trying to ask for my phone, but she just kept saying that I couldn't talk because of the tube. I asked for a pen and paper using hand signals. She brought them to me and after multiple attempts, I was able to write hallway legibly enough for her to read. I was able to ask for my phone to listen to music because it calms me down.

All I could think about was Paul. How he must be feeling sitting there by himself, dying with an incurable cancer alone. My heart was breaking for him.

A girl from the labs came to draw blood. She explained that she had drawn blood from me last night and she remembered me. She told me a few things to help jog my memory. She told me that I had a line of people down the hallway waiting to perform tests on me! She was one of them. She recalled hearing the doctor calling Paul and letting him come in to say goodbye to me. He didn't think I was going to make it through the emergency surgery. I'm sitting here listening to her telling me about what happened to me like she's telling me a story about someone else.

The ER doctor is also the chief of surgery of the hospital. Dr. England had to perform emergency surgery on me because I was about to die. They had to do the surgery because my leg had Streptococcus Cellulitis. It was turning septic! The doctor from respiratory had to intubate me when I quit breathing in ER. I'm terrified hearing all of this. Did this really just happen to me? I felt like I was in some kind of horrible dream that I couldn't wake up from.

I just wanted to see Paul! I needed to know that he was OK. I wanted to see my sister just in case I didn't make it. She means more to me than she realizes.

The hospital was only allowing 1 visitor at a time still. Paul came that afternoon to see me. It was so nice to see his face. He looked older, more tired, and scared! We talked about what happened to me and shared stories. He was trying to help jog my memory some more.

He said he sat in the car for 9 hours! That's how long it took from the minute I went in to the ER, and after the surgery, Since it was so early in the morning, Paul had to go home because they wouldn't let him in to see me.

Paul confirmed what the girl from the lab told me. He said that I was in trouble when I sent him the picture of me spitting up blood! We were both scared and crying. Neither one of us were out of the woods as far as our health.

Paul had spoken to Becky while I was in surgery, and again afterwards telling her I needed her to come see me. We were both tired, and I definitely needed rest, so I told him to go home and try to get some rest. I turned on YouTube on my phone and listened to "Until Then" until I fell asleep crying my eyes out. I wanted to be home with Paul taking care of him. Dear God, why is this happening to us? I felt so helpless.

Today is September 4th, 2020. I've been in ICU for 2 days now. I still have no idea what my leg looks like under all those bandages. I noticed blood leaking through in a couple of spots in my bandages. What in the world has happened to my leg?

The nurse got me up to sit in the chair. I didn't feel any pain. Either the pain medication was working well, or I just couldn't feel my leg. Not long after she left me in the chair, Becky came in to see me. I was so happy to see her I just busted out crying. I just wanted to keep hugging her. She didn't stay long but it seemed like a lifetime because I was so tired from losing so much blood. As I feel asleep, all I could think about was how much my Lil Sis loved me. She never came back to visit me after that. She has plenty of her own health issues and lived further away.

I had a drainage tube coming out of my thigh that I could see. I had an IV port in my neck with 6 IV tubes! I had 3 IV's in my arms and hand! They were loading me up on the strongest antibiotics and pain medicine! They had me on heparin so I wouldn't have another stroke! I have to take blood thinners for my heart, and since it was an emergency surgery, my INR level was way above the safety zone.

The nurse said that my doctor was coming in today to change my bandages! This should be interesting to see. Once he took them off and I saw it for the first time, I wasn't sure if I was going to vomit or pass out! I was cut from about my ankle to mid-calf! There was a deep hole in my lower leg, and it was packed with sterile surgical pads! He had to take them out, clean it out, and repack it. Damn, it hurt like hell! I had to turn my music on before he could touch me again! They would all begin to understand that it was the only thing that would calm me down so that they could take care of it!

All I could think about was how I needed to be braver than I had ever been in my life so I could get to go home and take care of Paul. He needed me so badly now. It was beginning to really mess with my mentality! It was already a mess because of Covid and his cancer.

Then, the top of my leg was cut maybe two inches from my knee halfway up my thigh! It was terribly bruised, and it hurt. It was so swollen and both areas were completely stapled shut! The pictures I took almost looked like a fake leg. I couldn't begin to tell you how many tests were done on me! The doctor kept wanting me to get an ultrasound done on it, but the bandages and changing it hurt bad enough, I couldn't imagine them going up and down my leg with that. Plus, the big hole in my leg! What if the gel got in there?

But, September 12th, my doctor begged me to have it done against my better judgement. The lady started at the top of my leg and every time she pushed, it hurt like hell! I just kept trying to concentrate on my music.

Now I'm really scared because she's getting ready to start on the bottom. Damn it hurts! I kept telling her how badly it was hurting but she just kept doing it. She was too busy watching the videos of Zulle Erna! But it was just too much, and I made her stop the testing.

I couldn't look at my leg. I was too scared. She, on the other hand, did and quickly wrapped a towel around it and called for transport to come get me. I was crying uncontrollably because of how bad it was hurting.

Paul was waiting for me when I got back to my room. He had brought Taco Bell for Sunday Night Football. It was the first game of the season and we both had been looking forward to it.

The guy from transport almost puked when my nurse took the towel off my leg!

My nurse immediately called Dr. England. The ultrasound gel had burned my leg! The skin had cracked open at the bottom and stuff was oozing out of it. The look of horror on Paul's face was so sad. I can only imagine what my face looked like. The entire surgical team came to my room! My nurse said she had never seen them get there fast on any patient before. She said I must be special to them for as fast as they got to my room. They hung out with us, watched a little bit of the game. They advised my nurse to leave my leg unwrapped for a while before putting the bandages back on. She was the only nurse who hugged me and let me cry on her shoulders. Her name was Rose, and I was blessed to have her as my nurse. I never saw her again.

September 15th, I got to go home. I couldn't wait for Paul to get there and take me home. You would think with everything I'd been through the doctor would have given me more than 10 pain pills! I would have nurses coming to the house to take care of me 3 times a week. They would have to change my bandages and monitor my INR levels and make sure I had everything I needed. But on the days that they didn't come I would have to do it by myself. Even cleaning out the hole in my leg! That was so painful, and I dreaded having to do it! But I had to be a "good soldier" so I could take care of Paul. That's how it felt to me, like I was a soldier because of how strong I needed to be.

Paul had Tony bring the potty chair up from the basement because there was no way I was going to be able to climb the stairs. I slept on the loveseat because it was the only place, I was comfortable at. Paul slept on the couch when he did sleep that is. He went days without sleeping due to his pain medication. We just watched over each other the best we could.

It would take several months for me to recover from my leg. Multiple visits from in home health care, and the surgical team. The burn from the ultrasound gel will never fully recover because it was considered a chemical burn! To this day it's still very red and painful! The scars will be a permanent reminder of the hell we went through. I'm forever grateful that God spared my life so that I could take care of my husband who was going through his own hell!

Chapter 10

A Turn for the Worse

Paul's sleep pattern was getting so out of control. He would sit up for days falling asleep with his PS4 controller in his hands, or about to fall off the couch. It was damn near impossible to get him to go to bed. But once he was in bed, he'd sleep for hours, sometimes days. I would tiptoe around the house so as not to wake him up. It would be great that he was finally resting, but it sure was lonely for me. You would think that I would use that time to get some rest myself, but no, my mind wouldn't shut down. Especially after the dreams I was having. Instead, I took that time to try to relax, process the day and my thoughts before it gets too overwhelming, and I just had a total breakdown. I remember reading a poem called "Silent Cry". I became the master of silent crying. At times, it felt like my chest was going to explode! I would just sit there in a daze, unable to absorb anything at times.

In the meantime, Paul was still waiting for his unemployment, and he's been waiting what is going on a year, and he wasn't receiving the added Covid pay which he desperately needed. We haven't made a house payment in months. Jason sent Paul some money to help catch up on the payments. Before I was able to go make the payment, the sheriff showed up with eviction paperwork! The credit union wanted it back.

I took the payment to them, and they gladly accepted it. It was basically every penny that we had to catch it up to date. So, we're thinking everything is fine, but nope. God had other plans for us. When I went the following month to make the house payment, they refused it. It was for the best anyways with our health, so it was time to start looking for a place to live. The weather sure wasn't being very cooperative starting the new year of 2021. We had multiple rounds of snow, 7-10 inches each storm mixed with bitter cold. It was all we could do to keep Paul warm. He's lost so much weight that he really felt the cold weather deep in his bones. The last thing he needed was to get sick.

Paul had a visit in February with Dr. Sapp. When Kim, the nūrse, weighed him, he only weighed 132 pounds. Last year he weighed over 200 pounds. He was having a lot of pain in his stomach, so she ordered an endoscopy and colonoscopy. The doctor has a rather long name that is hard to pronounce, so everyone called him by his first name, Chike. He performed the procedures on February 16th, 2021. He said he removed a polyp from Paul's stomach and sent it to be screened for cancer. Which the results confirmed. Less than a week later, while I went to the store at the top of the hill, Paul's sugar level dropped to 53! I needed to get some sugar in him quickly. I started buying glucose pills in case it happened again, which it did multiple times.

The best news came from March 19th when his unemployment finally went in the bank. It was truly a blessing especially since we had to move. Unfortunately, the good news didn't last long when an MRI showed that he now had cancer growing in his brain! We kinda wondered if he didn't have something going on up there because he was having memory issues.

One day, Paul was counting money, and he stopped several times, sometimes looking at it like he didn't know what it was. It was devastating to both of us. Paul had always been one of the smartest men I'd ever known and to see him like this totally broke my heart.

Trying to find a place to live wasn't easy. Either there was nothing available, or we didn't qualify. We were beginning to lose hope when we found two places that were available

I went to Andover apartments in Taylor Mill. The manager was a sweet lady, her name was Darlene. I was completely honest with her about our situation. She was sympathetic, especially since she had lost her husband to cancer as well.

Grief Before Death: A True Love Story

She showed me an apartment on the 2nd floor. I was so out of breath I could barely talk to her. My breathing hasn't been right since I had to be intubated. She noticed how hard it was for me to breathe and suggested we find an apartment on the first floor. We continued searching and becoming more and more anxious about everything. Paul was becoming so depressed and afraid to leave me alone when he passed away. He knew that I wouldn't really have anyone to be there for me. He asked Tony and Jason to look out for me.

Finally, a ray of sunshine and prayers answered. Darlene called from Andover apartments with great news. Our background check was back, and everything was good and ready to go. She had a 2 bedroom on the first floor with the laundry room right next to us. She said she would be there for me all the way through, and after.

She said "it's not just a place to live. God brought you to me and I'll help you." I just cried, feeling so blessed.

April 23rd, Paul was having another endoscopy at St. Elizabeth looking for more cancer. Once he was released, we went home to rest before we had to go to Andover. We needed to pay our deposit, 1st month's rent, get our keys and go over the lease. Such a heavy weight lifted off our shoulders. Paul was becoming more and more emotional each day, going from one extreme to the other. I wasn't sure how to help him except to not let him push me away. I assured him no matter what, I said until "Death Do Us Part", and I keep my word. I can only love him harder than I ever have.

We finally got moved into our new apartment and was beginning to get used to it. Then, a thought crossed my mind leaving me in tears. Our New Home would be his Last Home! Dear God, I cried, I've brought my husband here to die! Dear God help me please, was all I could manage to say.

Paul was using the Libre 2 for monitoring his sugar level which was staying more on the lower side these days. When he was able to urinate, it was really dark. He's lost so much weight he reminded me of a "human skeleton"! I'm sure that must sound morbid, but it's the gospel truth. He barely eats anything and sometimes he pukes it back up.

This is really beginning to break us down, physically, mentally, and emotionally. The only thing that kept us going was upcoming events like Isiah graduating, our 18th year wedding anniversary, birthdays, holidays, etc. we did our best to make each day count, sharing plenty of prayers and tears daily. Paul was mainly thinking about me more than himself. It was breaking his heart to think about leaving me behind in this cruel world. He knew that I wouldn't have anybody to love me like he did. I don't have many friends, but my best friend Rochelle was there for me even if it was just a text or something like that. That's what a friend does for you, be there for you throughout whatever type of day. I couldn't ask for a better friend than her.

June 2021, we lost my uncle Manley. I went to visit him in hospice on June 17th. It was heartbreaking to see him like that. He's always been my favorite uncle and I was going to miss him terribly. My heart broke for my Aunt Judy. They've been together forever, and this is going to be so painful for her. She's my favorite aunt and my dad's last remaining sister.

July 15th, we saw Dr. Sapp for follow-up on how the new chemo pill was working. It unfortunately had the same effects as the others, so he quit taking it in May! He actually gained 21 pounds and actually had an appetite again.

July 29th, Paul was having another endoscopy done. We were praying for good news but that wouldn't be the answer we would get. Dr. Chike told us that he found a polyp and removed it. I just broke down crying. Paul said "Don't cry, baby. We both know what it is!" Dear God, how many areas is it going to attack? The results confirmed that it was cancer.

August 23rd is our 25th Anniversary as a couple. I wanted it to be nice for him, he deserved it. I made an Anniversary wreath for us, blew up balloons, bought a cake and we ordered dinner out. John came over and had dinner with us. Paul wasn't feeling well so it was an early night for him. We cut our cake, holding hands. It was a first for both of us. We didn't eat any of it for two days!

August 31st, we saw Dr. Sapp again. She was still trying to convince him to start taking the chemo pills again because they were running out of options. Again, he refused. As far as his appetite went, he at least had an appetite. He asked me to leave the room so he could talk to her in private. When he walked out of her office and went to make a follow-up appointment, he was rather pale looking. I didn't ask any questions although I wanted to. I gave him his space until he was ready to talk to me about it. When we got to the car, he told me that he had asked her what she thought was going to kill him. She told him it would be his stomach. She said that the cancer could eat through, and he could bleed to death! We cried all the way home and most of the night.

Theresa kept trying to get us to come to Texas for a visit. She didn't quite understand just how badly he was doing until Tony explained it to her. She decided to come here to surprise him, but we had to pick her up from the airport so that wasn't going to work. She stayed for a week in total, a few days with us and a few days with Tony. We went to Sam's Club, and she got us all a bunch of food and such. It was really nice having someone to talk to in person and understand what we were going through. She was here for the test results and saw me always crying. Paul told her we do a lot of that these days. I cried when she went home, but nothing good lasts forever, does it?

Two weeks later, we found out that Paul had a new growth in his left cerebella hemisphere since June! This wasn't what we wanted to hear. When I first met him, he didn't believe a whole lot as far as the supernatural went. But, with facing a "Death Sentence" he was beginning to believe in it more. He was watching shows on YouTube about people dying and coming back to life. But September 2th, I'm not sure what was going on with us except we both were having strange dreams. My dream was bout black wolves with a black wolf puppy. Whoever saw the puppy got attacked by the adult wolves. When I asked Google about it, it said that to dream of a black wolf means the death of someone close to you. Paul dreamed about an alligator biting his arm but wouldn't do the death roll; nobody would help him. To dream of an alligator means betrayal by someone you think cares about you, but it's all a front! Strange dreams are an understatement.

We ordered a hospital bedside table so he could just stay in bed and eat. He's lost so much weight, and he stays so cold. To ensure he doesn't get sick, he needs to be where it's warm. He has his own little heater to keep him warm. Unfortunately, I would get so hot, I'd have to go to another room and open the window. I bought some serving trays and would carry our food to our bedroom so we could eat together. Then, I started pushing the food on the cart I use for laundry. It was so much easier, and I was always exhausted.

Paul was scheduled for an MRI on October 28th. The stuff he had to drink was making him feel sick. When they got him back there for the procedure, he puked. Then to have to lay on the table hurt him so badly they couldn't finish it. It was the first time I had to push him in the wheelchair. They were going to look for cancer in his hip again!

We saw Dr. Sapp again on November 11th. She ordered 3 more MRIs which he didn't want again. The brain scan results showed that the one they'd found earlier was still growing, and a new growth in the area was now affecting his spine.

Paul hated seeing me struggling to take care of him; it broke his heart, and he would cry about it. He tried to help with bringing groceries in until one day it was all he could do to life them up on the counter because he his hands were shaking too badly. He said, "It sucks knowing your strength is gone." We both had pretty good arm muscles but now his were totally gone. My heart kept breaking for him.

Then, on December 11th, Kentucky was hit with tornadoes! I knew we were going to get bad weather. I'm a weather freak and I wanted to be awake when the storms came through, but I fell asleep hard. I woke up with blinding lights in my eyes. I wasn't sure where I was. I got up to go in the other room and was walking on top of something. Wow. I guess we got some kind of weather because the curtain rod, the wall hinges, and the curtains were just laying on the floor! Damn, what the hell happened?

Paul said that he'd sat up for a while and it was getting pretty rough outside. Then, the power went out and he fell asleep. He wasn't sure what happened after that until I woke him up. A tornado in December? This world has gone insane.

Christmas was just around the corner, but this year was going to be different in many ways. We usually just buy our gifts and go ahead and give them to each other. But this year, we were going to wrap them and give them to each other on Christmas Day. We still picked out our gifts, but when they were delivered, we put them up for Christmas Day. It would probably be his last Christmas! What a horrible thought, but it was what was on both of our minds.

Chapter 11

Dead People

As 2021 ends, we had no idea what 2022 would bring us. We prayed for a better year with less growth of his cancer.

Paul was trying the chemo pill again, and over the 24 hours since, he already feeling like he'd lost his appetite. They can cause tears in the stomach lining and decrease the appetite! Already puking! And this was only the second of January! We saw Dr. Sapp again on January 11th, 2022. It was bad enough that he was feeling worse since taking the pills, but now she was telling us that the cancer was still growing in his lungs and adrenal gland! Again, she tried to convince him to take the pill because we were running out of options!

We were both so exhausted constantly. We decided on January 14th to take a much-needed nap. As I was laying there trying to go to sleep, I kept noticing shadows or something else. They were black, and oddly shaped. They're circling about the bed and there's several of them. They circle, swoop down towards Paul and then fly away. They remind me of the dementors in the Harry Potter movies! I notice his breathing is a little different, a little louder sounding than normal. When I tell him about it, he didn't sleep the rest of the weekend. He said, "I wish you would never have told me that!"

As if that wasn't bad enough, Paul is starting to hear voices again! People were calling his name. Voices he didn't recognize. Now, he's gone the entire weekend with no sleep. Plus, we're expecting snow. I don't drive in the snow, and his driving scares the hell out of me. We have an early appointment on January 17th for another brain scan. The brain scan results shows the tumors are still growing. It's so sad watching him. It's hard for him to concentrate, get up and walk around, especially coming back into our apartment. Although it's only four steps, he has nothing to grab onto. Therefore, he literally crawls on his hands until he's done with the steps. And then uses the wall to be able to get to a standing position again. I had to send a message to the doctor on February 12th because Paul's belly was really hurting, and he was having trouble urinating. That's not good, considering he only has the one kidney. She suggested another CT scan, pain meds, and rest. He had an appointment February 24th, which wasn't a good visit. The CT scan showed minor enlargement of a new mass in the adrenal gland! When asked about his pain level, it was a four out of five! That's even with his prescribed pain meds, which consisted of Oxycodone and morphine.

Paul and I have such an intense love for music, and we'd listen to it often. We would play songs for each other and cry, holding each other. He was so afraid to go to sleep, afraid he wouldn't wake up. He was afraid of the dead people talking to him! He was terrified of what was going to happen to me once he was gone. He didn't want me to commit suicide, so he made me promise that I wouldn't. Even as I'm writing this, I regret making that promise. I knew I'd go to hell, and I wouldn't be with him and that was my main thought, plus I made other promises I had to fulfill.

In our talks, he would cry, telling me how much he knew that it was coming. I asked him how he knew that, and his reply was because "I can feel it," and the dead people were telling him so! I can't imagine how terrifying that must have been for him. He told me about the train ride; when I asked him about it, he said "I was on a train with other dead people, but nobody would talk to me?" How heartbreaking it was hearing the stories about the dead people. Were they good or bad? Did they mean to cause any harm to him? Why wouldn't they talk to him? Questions that will always haunt me because there are/were no answers or explanations.

Paul's always been a kind, loving man, but at times it was like he was going out of his way to be mean to me. Was he trying to push me away in hopes it wouldn't hurt so bad? He would get short with Tony and sometimes Theresa too. I had enough one day. I was beyond tired and wasn't feeling my best and he was in rare form. I told him "You can be mean to me as much as you need to, but it's not going to change anything as far as my feelings go!" He broke down crying, asking me to sit by him on the bed. He just held me, and we cried forever, it felt like. Dear God, please wake us up from this horrific nightmare. We felt so humbled and broken. But we never gave up on our faith, regardless of what we faced. We knew it was in God's hands, God's plan.

I like being crafty and writing poems, and journaling. I saw down on March 6th in the living room while Paul and Tony played PlayStation 4 and I wrote Paul a poem. I titled it Grief Before Death. They yelled for me to come hang out with them and I took it with me to read it to him. He just cried when I finished reading it. He thinks it deserves to be published. He said I should write another one about cancer patient rights and being treated with dignity.

I don't know what we would have done without Tony always being here for us and with us. Anything we needed; he'd do it for us. Every spare minute he had; he'd spend it with us. There were times he would come over and Paul would be sleeping. That gave me time to tell him things he didn't know. It was killing both of us watching the man we love and admire succumb to his illness! God gives us strength and understanding.

It seems like these days, every doctor's appointment and the never-ending test results are going to lose. Now he has to see a brain surgeon. Paul said, "No matter what, don't let them cut into my brain!"

We saw Dr. Curry on February 2nd for a consult. Paul is already beyond anxious, and then to sit there waiting patiently for almost an hour, it's really testing his patience. He didn't appreciate what little bit of time he had left sitting in a waiting room. I've never seen him so angry! I just kept trying to keep him calm, and explaining how important it was to keep this appointment. Finally, Dr. Curry came in. He went over Paul's brain scan history and treatments. He suggested having another scan done in a couple of weeks, then a follow-up visit. We were so glad to be done with that appointment.

Since Paul had a MyChart account, we would see the test results the next morning. I always got up early because I took my morning medicine at 5 a.m. Test results were usually there by at least 6:10 a.m. So, I stayed awake to read them, praying for good news. I would just sit there, crying my eyes out, trying to be as quiet as possible. I was trying my best to be strong for Paul, but I'm only human. I hated breaking down in front of him. He looked to me for strength and I've never felt so helpless in my life!

The brain scan showed more growth and it's only been a couple of weeks! God, I don't want to tell him this. I pray he can catch a break just one time and get good news for a change. Needless to say, after the first visit with Dr. Curry, and the test results, neither of us were in a hurry to go back. We didn't wait as long as the last time, which was a good thing because Paul's nerves were shot. Dr. Curry showed us the areas it was growing in, and how radiation wasn't an option. Surgery was out of the question as well. We were standing beside each other when Dr. Curry said because of his health and the new growth, Paul's time frame was two months! I busted out crying and thought I was going to pass out. Paul grabbed hold of me so I wouldn't fall, and he was crying, too. The look on Dr. Curry's face was sad. He apologized for having to be honest like that, but that was Paul's diagnosis. This was March 2nd. He suggested considering hospice. That was our last time seeing him.

Paul would be seeing Dr. Sapp, or her Associates, weekly now, and doing chemotherapy afterwards. Paul would get so aggravated waiting for someone from chemo to come get him. We would spend three and a half to four hours between labs, Dr. Sapp, and chemo. Paul had been telling Dr. Sapp how anxious he had become, and sometimes she'd ask him if he was anxious. But she never offered him anything to help him. But what was coming next would change her mind. And the dead people kept talking to him.

Chapter 12

Beginning of the End

And the dead people kept talking to him!
At times, he had a scared expression on his face, or be really anxious. He said, "they keep calling my name." I asked if he was right with God. He believes he is, but was considering having Brother John, the pastor from my Aunt Judy's Church come pray with him. I have met him several times and Paul met him at Uncle Manley's service.

I finally talked Becky into coming for a visit on April 11th. It would be the first time I saw her since 2020! It was so nice to see her, I cried. We sat and caught up on things while Paul slept. It wasn't long before we heard him on the baby monitor. Paul had been telling people his "goodbyes", so I wasn't sure what was going to happen when we went back to visit.

When the cancer started, Paul weighed 235 pounds, and now barely weighs 130! At times, it was so hard to see him under the covers. He had become so anorexic, as the doctors described him! Becky wasn't sure what to do or say when we walked in there. She tried to joke with Paul by asking where the rest of him was? Paul replied, "yeah, there's not much left of me is there?" she told him she didn't want him to go anywhere. He tried to assure her that he was doing his best to stay. She lost it and started crying, which caused a chain reaction because we were all crying then. Paul gave her a big hug and told her "I'm not done fighting." He told her that I was going to need her, and he wanted to make sure that she'd be there for me. She told him she would be.

We have an appointment with Dr. Sapp today, April 13th. Paul had a CT scan done on his stomach and the results weren't good. The spot on his adrenal gland was increased! She suggested seeing Dr. Shah in Radiology. Paul again told her how anxious he had become, and still no reply. She'd been writing in MyChart how anxious he'd become but offered no help for him. I took the opportunity and asked if she could give him something for his nerves because every little noise made him jump, plus he was a nervous wreck. She finally agreed and wrote him a prescription for Valium. Finally, maybe he can be a little more comfortable.

Dr. Sapp says she believes it's getting close and maybe we should consider bringing hospice in. We knew it was coming, but to actually hear her say it shocked us. We weren't prepared for that. It hurt both of us terribly and those words became stuck in our heads the rest of the day. She noticed how badly he was feeling and cancelled treatment. She was going to call in Palative care! I asked her about a time frame, but she couldn't answer that question. She doesn't like the way it was in his brain. She's stopping treatment altogether and focusing on his quality of life. He's scheduled for another brain scan on April 26th.

We always watched a show called "Deadliest Catch" on Tuesday night. He was sleeping and I was trying to be quiet so he could get some much-needed rest. My body was tired and hurting, so I stretched out on the couch to watch it, but I fell asleep instead. I woke up hearing him coughing on the monitor. I heard him walking down the hallway, he was walking very slowly and staggering. He said he was lightheaded and dizzy.

We assumed it was his sugar, but it was good so what's going on? Paul said he felt like he needed to puke, but nothing came up. He said his ears were ringing really badly. His urine was dark and had a strong odor. He got his water and went back to bed with me right behind him.

We had an appointment with Dr. Shah on April 15th to discuss radiation treatments and his recent CT scan. He explained just how risky the treatment would be on the adrenal gland because of all the other organs around it. He suggested we take a couple of days, think about it, talk it over and let him know our decision. All I can think about was Dr. Shah saying, "one wrong move would be extremely dangerous!" Time was of the essence, so they scheduled an appointment for measurements. Everything had to be 100% precise.

Up until a couple of weeks previously, Paul had never mentioned how he'd always wanted a cowboy hat and a pair of boots. I wanted him to have whatever he needed or wanted. We looked together and he picked out the hat he wanted, and I ordered it. It was in the mailbox when we got home from seeing Dr. Shah. He was so excited and happy! That's what mattered to me, seeing his beautiful smile. It looks so good on him. A ray of sunshine in our gloomy world.

Easter was just a couple of days away and I wanted Paul to have a nice day. I fixed all his favorite foods in hopes he'd eat. Tony came over and had dinner with us. Paul loved the deviled eggs I made; said they were the best he'd ever had. Made my day to get a compliment like that, especially from him. He wasn't easy to cook for, and I'd hold my breath waiting for his opinion on the meals I cooked. He ate really well, and actually sat on the couch for a little while. He did really good until he started hurting and needed to go lay down. "God bless your soul" I told him and cried.

The radiation treatments were heavy on our minds. So many risks to consider. So many things could go wrong. Was it worth the risk? I can honestly say I didn't want him to do it. Everything inside me said it wasn't a good idea! I was absolutely terrified. But he decided to at least try and see what happened. He still had fight and determination, and he planned on fighting until there was no fight left.

Paul's appointment for measurement was April 19th. The radiation department had to get everything just right because one wrong move would have dire consequences. Paul had lost over 100 pounds and stayed cold all the time. He would wear two shirts. When he went back, they had him take his shirts off and get on the table. When he was done and came to the car, he told me how embarrassed he was for everyone to see his bones. The nutritionist said he was severely underweight, and he was also losing muscle. He was literally down to the bones. Paul said that laying on the table hurt him really badly. We just sat in the car crying. I was just to upset to drive for a few minutes. We came home and he took his pain meds, and we took a nap.

Paul had made a "to-do list" for Tony and me. He waited until we were all together to show it to us. Paul said he wanted us to do our best to get it done before he passed away. We just sat there crying our eyes out. Paul told us he knows it's coming but he was going to hold on as long as he could. Paul told us he didn't want to leave us. It was killing all of us.

Ever since the beginning of 2022, he'd been having to wait every time for the refills on his pain meds. It's been like that since the beginning of the year!

Today is April 22nd. I called in his refill request yesterday. He wouldn't get his meds until April 28th! Unacceptable! How do you leave a cancer patient with no pain meds? He's having trouble breathing today. Tony came over after work for a while.

Paul's first radiation treatment on his adrenal gland is April 27th. We thought it was a practice run, but it was the real deal. I wasn't allowed to go back with him, so I had to sit in the car, and I talked to Jamie on the phone. Before we went, Paul said he wasn't feeling right. He'd been so stressed out lately over everything. He says he's lightheaded and he's staggering! Paul's brain scan says he has a new one on the right side! When we got home, we laid down and took a nap. I must have really been tired because I was asleep as soon as my head hit the pillow.

I woke up to a banging sound and him yelling for me. I wasn't sure where he was at first. We had fallen asleep with the TV on, and it was blaring! He was sitting in the bathroom and hitting the counter with the plunger to get my attention. He said his head was busting, he's never hurt so bad in his head before! He's puking and can't get off the toilet. He's been hurting for a few days now. He remembers going in the radiation and coming out but everything else is a blur. We stopped at Burger King on the way home, but he never ate! Paul took some of his Oxycodone and passed back out. I went in the middle bedroom so I could smoke and still be close to him. Dr. Sapp called. I assumed it was in regard to the message I left, but she hadn't seen it yet. She told me about his brain scan, not realizing Dr. Shah had already told us. It was the one and only time she ever called us. I informed her of what was going on with him, and she instructed me to keep a watchful eye on him and take him to the ER if necessary. She says she thinks it's time for hospice.

Paul was sick all night, his head still hurting and he's still puking. He asked me to cancel treatment today. The radiation team wasn't very happy about it, but I don't know what to tell them. I think he's had a stroke. His face is drooped on one side, his speech is slurred and his head is hurting so bad. At least he quit puking. But then again, he hasn't eaten anything in over 30 hours, either! Paul's radiation treatments were scheduled from April 27th to May 2nd.

Paul says he's losing his fight, he can feel it coming. He told me out of the blue one day that God was guiding him through, and it wasn't so bad. Paul told me to never be afraid of dying because God is there to help you every step of the way to come home. He said he was another step closer to going down the rabbit hold. We just held each other crying.

Chapter 13

Going Down the Rabbit hole

Paul's health is declining more and more each day. We're all afraid of losing him but we can all see it happening. He wants me by his side constantly, which is exactly where I want to be. I don't even go to get my INR done or go to the store. Thankfully, he only has a couple more radiation treatments left. Paul has an appointment with Dr. Shah on May 2nd and a treatment afterward. I have an appointment with Dr. Diaz, but I'm going to cancel. Paul can't drive anymore, and our appointments are too close together. I wanted to be at his appointment to see if Dr. Shah thinks he's had a stroke. Paul has treatment and then we'll see Dr. Shah. I actually was surprised at what Dr. Shah had to say about the possibility of a stroke. Paul starts telling him about his first radiation treatment, what happened when we got home, and told him to take a good look at his face. Paul told him about his hearing being a steady ringing in his ear and how his vision was changing. Dr. Shah looked at his face for a couple of minutes, listened to him talk, and his speech was pretty slurred. Dr. Shah looks at him right in his face and tells him "You didn't have a stroke." He continues with, "The cancer did that to your face, but not a stroke." I thought to myself *"are you for real?"* I mean, it's only obvious he's had a stroke. I've had two myself, and I watched my dad die having multiple strokes. We came home, both of us knowing unless you do a brain scan, you can't tell if there's bleeding going on up there!

We just sat and cried! He was saying how much everyone at the doctor's office and the medical staff had let him down. Paul said, "I'm just a guinea pig to them, a paycheck!" he had been put through the hoops and nothing helped. He again asked me to write a poem about how cancer patients should be treated with dignity and respect. He said that they shouldn't schedule so many appointments at the same time because your time on Earth was already being shortened by the cancer, and they were wasting the rest of it keeping them sitting in the waiting rooms. At least he can get some rest until May 4th. That was when his next appointment was with Dr. Sapp.

Paul's speech and balance are way off today. He's really not doing well today. Dr. Sapp noticed it and asked him what was going on with him. He explained everything to her, and that Dr. Shah said it wasn't a stroke. She remembered the conversation we had that day on the phone. She said it was time to bring Hospice in, and she was releasing him from oncology! It wasn't exactly what we expected her to say.

We were already crying, even the nurse was crying, but what Dr. Sapp said next floored us. She gave him a time frame of a few months! Later, she put her final notes in MyChart saying that Paul's brain is basically full, and he has fluid on it! Why couldn't she have told us that in person? We had to read it in MyChart. I've never seen a patient of any kind get treated the way Paul had been treated. I think we were in shock. We didn't know what to do. What to think? The only thing we need to do was love each other and cry together. We were going to have to tell Tony soon because he was on his way over to see us. It was hard for him to accept. It was hard for everyone to accept it when we explained everything to our families and friends. Needless to say, neither of us slept very well that night, so many thoughts going through our minds. We were trying to process what Dr. Sapp had told us as far as the time frame. How she couldn't tell us in person about his brain scan. He was getting worse throughout the night with the pain in his head and everything else. By morning, he was ready to go to the ER. Paul's always been a tough guy unless he's really bad, so going to the ER would be his last option, but he decided he needed medical treatment. Because of whatever is going on with him in his head, he feels "head heavy." When he tries going down steps, the weight of his head pulls him forward and he almost falls. I had to call John because Tony was working. We needed John to help Paul get down the steps and into the car, and into the ER. We told the receptionist that the cancer center had sent him, but we still waited for hours. John needed to leave so Tony came to the hospital and stayed the whole time. The ER doctor ordered a brain MRI, which showed acute hemorrhage and tumor combinations in the left cerebellum. He would be put on steroids for the swelling in his brain. Since he no longer had a doctor in oncology, the ER doctor reached out to Dr. Neil's office. He would look over his test results then call the ER to talk to Paul he explained to him that his new diagnosis was for bleeding brain metastasis. He was having a new weakness, he was now deaf in his right ear, and his eyelid was drooped, and it wasn't able to close. Dr. Neil explained that given his underlying diagnosis and plans to pursue hospice care, he recommended continued focus on his comfort. He also recommended against neurosurgical evaluation and future CT scans. Paul told Dr. Neil to code him to be DNR.

Tony and I already knew Paul's plans, but to hear him actually tell the doctor that made it seem so surreal. They admitted Paul and we waited until they came to get him before we left. Paul was released the next afternoon. He was basically sent home to die.

They've given up on him. They didn't know his determination though. You can see the tiredness in Paul's face. He keeps the TV so loud because of his hearing loss. He even tried using headsets, but it doesn't help. He tries playing Madden on PlayStation 4, but the way his eye is drooped he's having trouble reading it. He just sits in a daze. I wonder what he's thinking about. This is the hardest thing I've ever seen or went through. It hurts us beyond words!

Again, I asked him if he wanted to talk to Brother John. He said "yes, yes I would." I called Aunt Judy, and she called Brother John who was more than willing to come see Paul and pray with him, and for him. Aunt Judy and Brother John came over on May 8th. They had a really good talk while I showed Aunt Judy our apartment, and to give them time alone. Brother John prayed for and with Paul. Both of them thought they knew each other from somewhere. Paul totally redirected his life with God and was at peace with that. But, a few hours later, Paul wasn't at peace. His stomach hurt him all night long. He said it was like he needed to poop, and nothing happened. He was moaning so badly in pain; my heart was in pieces watching him hurt like this. I definitely needed help, so I called Tony. He was there immediately. Paul would get on the potty chair, and I'd rub his back hoping it would help, but it never did. I was glad when Tony got there so we could take turns rubbing his back. He was getting weak, and we were having to help him from the chair to the bed. After a few minutes he would want back on the chair. Still nothing happened. We thought maybe an enema would help, but it didn't. This went on all night. We couldn't take it anymore, seeing him in so much pain! We started telling him there was nothing we could do for him. Like it or not, he needed to go to the ER.

Paul is a very prideful man whose main concern was leaving a bunch of medical bills for me to have to worry about. That's why he wouldn't go to the ER. His pride almost cost him his life. Today is now May 9th, and he's agreed to go to the hospital. We had to call an ambulance because there's no way we can get him to the car. We follow the ambulance to the hospital and meet him in the ER. After doing paperwork, they allowed us to go back to be with him.

Once we got to the ER, the doctors examined him, and did CT scans to find out he has a "perforated bowel". They have to do emergency surgery ASAP! He was coded as critical. They were giving him massive pain meds and they weren't helping. I know who the doctor was even behind his mask, he was Dr. England. He was the same doctor who saved my life when that happened to my leg. We were both very comfortable he would be taking care of Paul. He recognized me as well. I told him it was "God's Plan. Now you have to save his life like you saved mine." He reassured me he would. The surgery seemed to take forever. Tony and I went and got something to eat and to our house. We were a mess! We were terrified of losing Paul. It was breaking our hearts and souls to watch him suffer.

Finally, surgery is over, and Paul is in recovery. Dr. England came out to talk to us and said Paul had a hole in his small intestine, and he cut it off and repaired it. However, there's more cancer there. Which means it could happen again. The treatment plan was hospice and comfort care. At least he looks peaceful after last night.

We go visit him the next day, May 10th. He's so tired and in a lot of pain. We didn't stay long because he needed to rest.

May 12th is a horrible day for me so far! I'm beyond exhausted and I feel like I'm walking around in a fog. I took half of a Xanax last night for anxiety and sleep. Thankfully Paul understands. He says I don't have to hurry. He's wanting the tube out of his throat, but he has to tolerate a liquid diet first which he does. However, the nurse forgets to text the doctor to let them know that. When Eric, Dr. England's associate comes in and I told him, he takes the tube out. Paul is so happy. Eric took the nurse out into the hall. I'm guessing she's in trouble for not texting them, because she never came back in the room.

May 13th, and he's still in the hospital. If he can go to the bathroom, he can go home. He says it sounds like an airplane landing in his deaf ear, and a man and a woman talking in the other. I wrote on his patient board that he's deaf, but the nurses don't pay any attention to it. He says he sees people who aren't there. He said he doesn't want to sleep in the middle bedroom where the hospital bed is. We had set that room up for him when he would need it. He doesn't want to spend his last day's sleeping alone.

Paul said now the dead people are poking him like they're seeing if he's still alive. He said when he moves, they go away, but come back later.

May 14th, he finally gets to come home. They released him without him having a bowel movement! That was what Dr. England was waiting for. They treated him horribly, St. Elizabeth did. It wasn't Dr. England or any of his staff, they were good to Paul. Tony brought Paul home and straight to the bed. They had brought a wheelchair for us to be able to help him move around easier in case of emergencies. He slept the rest of the day.

May 15th, Paul's mind is half gone! He doesn't remember they sent him home to die! He's aggravated and wants to argue with me. I'm exhausted and he's wide awake. I make out a full day menu, that way he can choose what he wants to eat but his stomach hurts. He's slipping further and further into the rabbit hole.

Chapter 14

Not Even Death Can Keep Us Apart

May 17th, 2022, the hospice team came today! This has to be a bad dream, please wake me up from this nightmare. They set up his medications and brought paperwork for us to sign. John stopped by and Paul explained to him that he was at that point where it could happen anytime. The only thing that I'm supposed to do is to call hospice. John's having a hard time processing everything, we all are. I sat by Paul all night in the dark, watching TV and being quiet. But, as soon as night came, he was wide awake, and I was ready to go to sleep. I was afraid to go to sleep if he was awake in case he got up and fell.

Today is John's birthday. Paul and I had a long talk with him. Paul was aggravated and I had to explain to him that it was the steroids. He wants to get as much of his Madden game done as possible. But, since the stroke, he can barely see it to play it. John sat there and played PlayStation for him to get as much done as possible before he needed to leave. Tony was coming over as well.

May 21st, 2022. Paul is still struggling with his hearing and his eye. We're pretty sure that he's had another stroke. His eye won't close at all now! His face is more drooped, and his speech is worse. I set up arrangements with the funeral home today. None of this seems real! It's pouring rain and the thunder is really loud. He just about jumps out of the bed every time it claps. Dear God, please help him, I pray.

May 24th, 2022 today is our 19 year Wedding Anniversary. He had written in the calendar that he wanted to be here to celebrate it with his wonderful wife. Paul's hearing was totally gone now. He wrote on the top of the notebook paper "must write to me, I'm deaf!" how much more does he have to suffer? Please God, show him some mercy, I prayed.

Tony came over and wasn't sure what to think when he saw that. You can see the sadness in his face. I hurt for Tony, too. He's been right by our side from the minute we found out about the cancer! He told me several times, "thanks for taking care of and loving my brother." He said it was killing his soul watching him go, and he can't imagine what I must be going through. I told him I'd seen so many things I didn't want to see, and it would haunt me forever!

We didn't do a lot for our anniversary. We ordered some dinner from the restaurant and just hung out at home. Tony stayed for a while before he went home. At the end of the day, he wrote it in the calendar, "woohoo, I made it". He was really happy to be here, and with me by his side. He told me that he knew he had picked the right woman to be his wife and companion for his life.

May 25th, 2022, Paul has a hospice appointment this morning. She confirmed that he's had more strokes and that he is now on a "decline path." He's really not doing well today, and his breathing is bad. She suggested that we keep him as comfortable and stress free as possible. She said "talking to dead people" is a good thing because they're helping him through. She said, "He has one foot in this world, and one foot in the other!" Paul had been wanting food from Golden Corral; he loved their chicken. He asked Tony to pick him up several things from there since he was coming to see us. He actually ate pretty good, and we talked to Tony for a little while. We could tell Paul was getting tired and needed to get some rest. But right before Tony left, Paul's stomach was starting to hurt. I used the excuse of going to the kitchen to get a pop when in reality I was waiting for Tony to come out. That way, we could talk about our concerns better by ourselves. He said, "if his stomach starts hurting worse, or if you need me, I'll be home." I told him thanks and he left.

And it did get worse! Paul's stomach was acting just like it was before! He still had the staples in from his surgery! His pain level is 5 out of 5! His temperature is 99.1! He falls asleep for a few minutes and then he's right back awake hurting. I'm petrified! He could barely get back into the bed after trying to use the potty chair. I called Tony and he's on his way.

Paul asked me if I was ready to let him go. I told him "never." This went on the entire night! I fell asleep for a couple of hours, but I could still hear him moaning in pain, and Tony was trying to help him.

May 26th, 2002. Somewhere around 5 a.m., I went to make a cup of coffee. I could hear his moaning in the kitchen. I was furious! Why? Why does it have to be like this? Why does it have to be so painful? Praying that he didn't have to suffer anymore. I know Tony had to be exhausted. He'd been up with him all night to let me get some rest. I think we both knew that Paul's battle was coming to an end. He has a decision to make about treatment. I can't take it anymore seeing him hurt. I'm afraid that he's going to start bleeding in his stomach and bleed out.

I asked him if he wanted to go to the ER, or should I call Hospice? He said, "the surgery almost killed me to begin with, and I don't want to die there!" "I want you to do what I told you to do, call hospice!" "Dear God, I'm not ready to say goodbye to you," I cried as I called hospice. Within a couple of hours, hospice was here and talking to him through writing. They explained what the "comfort care" consisted of, and if he's sure he's ready. He nods his head yes, and they mention taking him to hospice! I told them "He's not going anywhere! He's exactly where he wants to be, and I have his living will to prove it!"

She said she was just making sure and started to give Tony and I instructions of how much, how often to administer the comfort meds. Then, she explained the time sheet, and how to fill it out. I'm hearing everything she's saying, but I'm in shock, numb, whatever you want to call it. This can't be real, can it?

Tony left shortly after hospice left to meet Jason at his house so he could come over to see Paul. We were advised to call the family in. After he left, I went back to be with Paul. We just sat there looking at each other, holding hands, hugging, and crying. No words were spoken, we didn't need them, we knew what each other was thinking and feeling. We were in our own little world, and it was such a painful place. The meds made him very sleepy, and he wasn't awake when Jason got there. I had written in the notebook earlier that he was coming. He cried. He hated leaving us all behind. He hated seeing the sadness on our faces. All the tears we cried. He assured me again God was with him and so were the "dead people". I know what's going on, OK? I got it! My everything is dying! And I'm helping him! But, in my mind, it's like I'm watching a movie, or reading a book. I'm not ready to accept it.

John came by later that night and brought us some Skyline chili. We were very grateful. He went back to sit with Paul. Paul kept trying to get up to urinate, and he wasn't strong enough to get up. I had to call hospice so they could put a catheter in.

We took turns sleeping. I had John wake me up every 4 hours so I could give Paul the medication. John left in the middle of the night. He had to work in the morning. Jason and Tony left early in the morning because Jason had to go to work also. I told Tony I'd be okay for a little while because hospice was coming to put the catheter in. He made it back before they got there.

Today is May 27th, 2022. The nurse said it was just a matter of time now. Was she really telling us this? I felt as if I was going to faint. I'm so numb. We would sit in there with him, talk to him, and I would continue giving him his meds. There was a part of me that felt like I was killing him. Committing murder. I had to keep reminding myself I was doing it just the way he asked it to be done. I was easing his suffering and letting him be free from his pain. I have to keep being strong for him.

We noticed at 6:03 pm that Pauls' breathing was becoming very heavy. Tony thinks it's close. I don't want to hear that, dear God, no! I called hospice to see if he was going through what they call "transitioning."

It was time for another dose of "comfort meds". Tony had seen me do it enough, so he offered to do it for me this time. Tony said it made him feel like he was killing him. I told him I had been feeling that way too, but

I know it's what he asked me to do, and it was helping him to not suffer anymore, and we both just cried.

I read him a poem for cancer patients called "Prayer for Relief." After I read it to him, I sat there crying, with Tony standing beside me. I remembered Aunt Judy telling me how Hospice said to let them know that it's okay to go, that you'll be okay, and how much you love them. I sat there holding his hands and telling him what Aunt Judy said to say. Tony told him the same thing. We had to walk away for a few minutes to compose ourselves. We went back a few minutes later to check on him. Paul's breathing is labored, and his eyes are fixed! Paul's left eye didn't close since the recent strokes, but they're fixed. I knew it was coming and called Jamie and Becky so they can see him one last time and say goodbye. I called John to tell him that he need to get here, but he didn't want to accept it. Tony had to call John and tell him if he wanted to say goodbye, he needed to get to the house.

Nobody knows when Death calls until it happens. We thought we had more time. We went to the middle bedroom to smoke and cry without him knowing. We were both being strong, just the way he wanted us to be. But inside, we were Broken!

Tony walked in to check on him, and I was coming right behind him when he yelled my name. My heart's pounding! I told Tony, "You better not be yelling because of why I think you're yelling!" Tony starts to cry and said, "he's gone!" I stood there for a second in disbelief, and then it hit me. I sat down in the chair before I fell down. I started crying and put my hands on top of his. And in that instant, it felt like a million pounds of weight came off of my shoulders, he's not in pain anymore was all I could think of. Tony said that he felt the same way. God has a very special Angel now, but we have holes in our hearts that can never be filled again. I am finally able to feel my legs and the rest of my body. I'm in shock. Knowing that Death is coming doesn't make it any easier, after all, Death! My mind start to work again, and I call Hospice. They're sending someone and calling the funeral home. I called Jamie at 9:26 and told her that "he's gone home." I sent messages to Rochelle and Becky. Tony walked outside to call John to see where he was. He was just pulling in. He could tell that something was wrong when Tony told him to meet him in the parking lot. John has trouble with death and anger issues. John's temper scares me to be honest. I wasn't sure what was going to happen? John's emotions were everywhere, needless to say.

We were all in our bedroom. I was sitting in the chair with my hands on top of Paul's. Tony and John were on the other side of our bed. Paul and I had been listening to a song by BLS called "Farewell Ballad" recently. I started to play it on my phone. I put my hand inside of his and he squeezed my hand and just held on. I gasped! Tony and John looked at me like I was crazy. I told them to look at our hands! They couldn't believe their eyes! We all started looking to see if he was breathing. Tony took his pulse and BP. There was none! I had John take a picture of it, and I told them "Not even Death can keep us apart!"

The nurse from Hospice came and went to the other side of the bed to check his vitals. She said she needed to come to my side of the bed and check his eyes. I motioned to our hands and told her that he won't let me go, you'll have to work around me. I didn't let go until the funeral home transport got there. I literally had to pull my hand out of his. I had told him that he had to take me with him when he went. He was supposed to put me in his pocket and take me with him. I didn't want to be in this world without him! But he made me promise that I wouldn't commit suicide so that we could be together in our next life. He promised me that he would never leave me, and he hasn't. He's in my heart, memories, and every once in a while, he lets me know it too, one way or another.

Epilogue

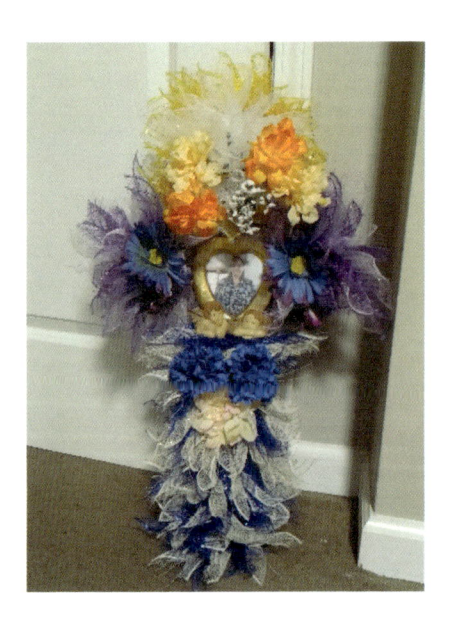

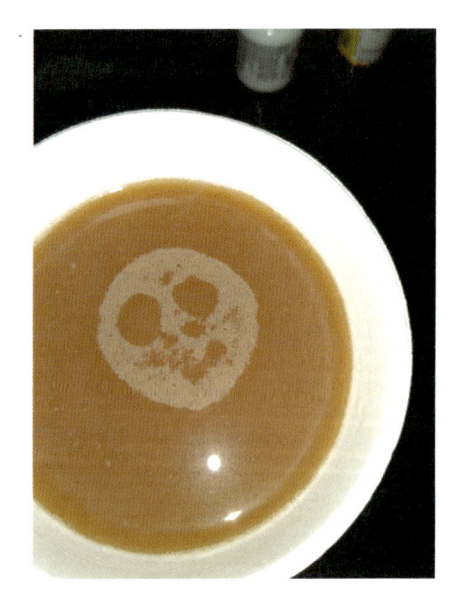

I knew that when I started writing "Our Story" it was going to be difficult, but until I started writing it, I had no idea just how hard it was going to be. So many emotions to deal with. So many memoires, some good, some bad. Remembering all the people I've lost and how much I miss them. But none of it hurt worse than saying goodbye to my husband, Paul. He truly was, and always will be, my Soulmate. We knew the kind of love other people only wish they could know. The kind you see in love stories, read about in books, or dream about. We were so "in tune" with each other, we could have a conversation without saying a word.

I'm grateful to have known Paul. He came into my life when I desperately needed someone there. I learned a lot from him, and he learned plenty from me. You have to be able to give in order to take! We definitely did a lot of giving and taking, but that helped us grow closer in so many ways. When I said in my wedding vows to him, the meaning of my "promises" to him were clear in my heart and mind. I never meant anything truer and more sincere in my life. But whoever thinks that when they're saying "until death do us part" how that was going to be? Did you ever think far enough into the future to think it would never happen to you? I didn't! I never dreamed that day would come that I'd have to go through it!

Between my age and my health, we both assumed that I would die before him. But God had other plans for us, and without His mercy, love, and guidance, we would never have completed our journey together, Until Death Do Us Part.

When I almost died in 2020, and the cancer diagnosis and Covid 19, I wanted to start "Our Story." I started making a timeline, going back through memories, messages, old calendars I had saved for years. I just kept adding more and more so one day, when I was ready, maybe I could actually start it. I want "Our Story" to be known.

Things are really lonely and painful without Paul. Walking the path of grief isn't a pleasant trip. But it helps knowing that he's still walking it with me, just like he said he would be.

Paul will always be in my heart, thoughts, and memories. Paul has let me know on numerous occasions that he is still with me, and no, I'm not crazy! I promise you I'm not.

I can give you plenty of examples of the signs he shows me. Like the day Tony and I were going over Paul's "to do" list, and there was a tornado in Goshen, Ohio. That's quite a way away from us, so it had nothing to do with our house in Kentucky, but our bedroom lights flickered several times whenever we said his name. The bedside radio clock doesn't reset itself to the correct time! I always had him reset it, but this time it reset itself! Or did it? I only know that when I fell asleep, I was going to have to reset it. I was going to try and figure it out, but I didn't have to because it somehow was on the right time when I woke up! It's never done that before.

I had to go to the Spectrum office to switch it to my name, but I wasn't sure where it was, so I was using GPS and my headset. I was at the light to either go straight or turn left which would have taken me to the hospital area where the cancer center is. Suddenly, I hear his voice in my headset saying, "hey" because I missed the turn.

The AC in our bedroom doesn't make beeping sounds by itself! The only time it makes noise is when you use the remote to adjust it! I was sitting in the living room, and I heard it through the monitor.

One night, I had a bad dream and the next morning, I made my coffee and sat down to make cigarettes. I was crying and I picked up my cup of coffee to get a drink and I literally about dropped it! There was a strange picture of a smiling face in my coffee! I definitely took a picture of it. Nobody I've shown it to knows what to think when I show it to them!

I truly believe "Our Story" hasn't ended. We believed that we really have known each other for many lifetimes, and we have many more to share. Ours is a True Love Story that never ends. I have to believe in that. It gives me the strength and purpose to keep his memories alive, and "Our Story" to be told. I hope that somehow "Our Story" will help others to deal with cancer, or whatever they might be facing, to never give up hope. I pray that you will be blessed to have known the type of love we had in life, and the kind of love we have in death. Love never dies! To you, Paul, I finish my book, all in Your Memory. My Love for you is Eternal, and one day, Paul, we will "Catch the Rainbow." Until then, my Darling.